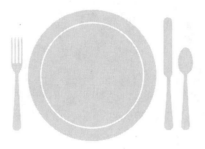

THERESA ALBERT

COOK Once a Week, EAT WELL Every Day

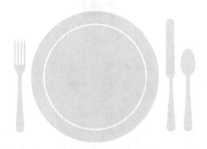

MAKE-AHEAD MEALS
that Transform Your Suppertime Circus into
RELAXING FAMILY TIME

MARLOWE & COMPANY

NEW YORK

COOK ONCE A WEEK, EAT WELL EVERY DAY:
Make-Ahead Meals That Transform Your Suppertime Circus into Relaxing Family Time
© 2005 by Thyme for Supper

Published by
Marlowe & Company
An Imprint of Avalon Publishing Group Incorporated
245 West 17th Street • 11th floor
New York, NY 10011-5300

AVALON
publishing group incorporated

Originally published as *Cook Once a Week* by HarperCollins Publishers Ltd in 2005.
This is a revised edition, published by arrangement.

Library of Congress Cataloging-in-Publication Data is available from the publisher.

ISBN-13: 978-1-56924-339-8
ISBN-10: 1-56924-339-5

9 8 7 6 5 4 3 2 1

Designed by Pauline Neuwirth, Neuwirth and Associates, Inc.

Printed in Canada

Dedicated to Guy and Jameson.
From my first disaster, Jerk Tofu, through breast milk, baby food, and Red River
Cereal, all the way to sushi for fireside supper—both of you tried every bite, gave
honest opinions, and gave me the courage to go on.

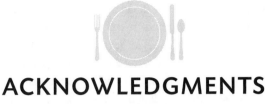

ACKNOWLEDGMENTS

No one could have predicted the amount of work necessary for this book to go from a seed of an idea for a business to a tree heavy with fruit. It takes a lot more than water and sunshine, and I owe thanks to a lot of people for their input and support. In utterly random order:

My mumnet group for keeping me alive in the early (and ongoing!) days of motherhood and for encouraging me, testing recipes (and buying this book!); my mom, Huguette, and her George, my dad, Ron, and my sisters, Michele and Cheryl for thinking I am weird and loving me anyway; my Cape Breton family, who turned out a fine brother-uncle-son and let him marry someone from away; Mercedes Rothwell for her skill in envisioning the prototype; Jeannie, Monica, and Linda for working with me in my "day job" and using these recipes over and over until we got them right; all the clients over the years who trusted us with their tummies; the dieticians and nutritionists who trusted us with their clients, especially Aileen Burford-Mason; Kirsten Hanson, who got an unsolicited prototype from an unknown and took a chance—you made me an author, thank you; Felicia Quon who got me the good gigs to promote this gem, Akka Janssen who called one fine afternoon to say she had a "nibble" in the U.S. which turned into one heck of a bite 48 hours later. The entire team at HarperCollins, who made me feel welcome and worthy; Hal Roth, Rosemarie Superville, and Paolo Cristante, who made the days in the photo studio fun and beautiful. My new American family at Marlowe, especially Kylie Foxx who made a good book even better with her pickiness and fantastic ideas.

To Donna Beck, Erin Booth, Mary Delli-Colli, and Babs Thurber, thanks for being awesome friends and "other moms" when I just could not be there for Jameson; the Keilhauers, the Viscas and the Bedards for being "chosen family"; Jackie Dais-Visca and Fiona Orr, who receive the award for best legal interpreters when reams of legalese make no sense; recipe testers, we all owe a lot to you; and all of the cooking class kids who try everything, teach me something every day, and have learned to say "It's not my taste" instead of "Ewwww." And to Matthew Gerrard who taught me, at 17, to "make a wish."

I owe the most thanks to my little family: my husband, Guy Ratchford, who saw the train coming and chose not to get off the tracks; he actually got on board my locomotive life and became the fuel that keeps me going. My daughter, Jameson, has been the impetus for everything: her birth set me on a path of motherhood, causing a career veer that led to this book. Trying to balance work and home may never have happened if not for her. She teaches me to be patient, kind, humble, and real—but she still has to eat her broccoli.

ACKNOWLEDGMENTS

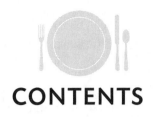

CONTENTS

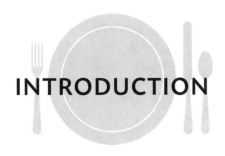

INTRODUCTION

*C*OOK *ONCE A WEEK, Eat Well Every Day* provides a revolutionary meal-planning system that will save you hours thinking about meals, grocery shopping, and the kitchen. It simplifies things by providing you with a meal plan for a workweek's worth of surefire family pleasers. Here's how:

- **Most recipes are designed to be successfully doubled and the balance frozen for future use.** Suggestions for making leftovers into brand-new meals (these are the Second Supper part of the recipes) are included to stretch three cooked meals into five—one for every night of the workweek.

- **Each weekly plan is designed to be cooked in three hours during one afternoon.** Using no more than a few hours on a Sunday, you can prepare not only that night's dinner but also the meals for the rest of the week. The economy of motion never looked so good. The idea is to get as much done as possible. If you have to be in the kitchen anyway, why not let it be the *only time* you lift or clean a pot all week!

- **All of your nutritional needs have been considered.** *Cook Once a Week, Eat Well Every Day* has no trans fats, lower starch and carbs (we use whole grains), lots of vegetables, and keeps healthy fats in healthy proportions. Although it is in no way intended to be a diet book, parents who are trying to watch their weight while also feeding their kids will be relieved of the struggle to do both at the same time without making two meals at every turn!

- **With detailed shopping lists,** *Cook Once a Week, Eat Well Every Day* **reduces the cost of preparing healthy family meals while making it**

easier to do so. Buying only what you need reduces the feeling-guilty cycle of buying with the best of intentions, letting things rot, then throwing them away. Our shopping lists include everything you need to get the job done (deliciously!) and nothing more. This is a much smarter way to shop.

We know that today's busy schedules have you running home for supper through the workweek, so we have provided for three nights of preplanned suppers and two nights of meals to assemble from the fruits of your earlier labors (they used to be called leftovers but we call them Second Suppers, because they're leftovers with a twist).

COOKING FOR, AND WITH, KIDS

ALL OF THE recipes in this book are based on a family of four, and you can scale up or down as needed. Kids under eight usually eat half portions, kids between the ages of eight and twelve can count as about three-quarter portions, and kids over twelve are anybody's guess from zero to two portions. You'll have to figure out the adolescent stomach as you go along—just like their clothes and music.

We have included an entire chapter of recipes for kids to make with you (see Bonus Kids Week). If you've got little ones, we suggest that this meal plan be your first foray into your new system for two reasons: the meals are utterly kid friendly and the recipes are the easiest of them all. Some families will use the Bonus Kids Week over and over again, venturing only into the other chapters when they have company or host a big family dinner. For fussy eaters, perhaps your best bet is to make these kids' meals and freeze everything in single-serving sizes. Kids can microwave them *only after they have tried the rest of what is put on the table*. No hassling or arguing; simply suggest that they get one of the meals that *they* made and microwave it. As long as your microwave oven is within reach, any child over three can do this—with supervision.

Our experience with kids tells us that they are much more likely to eat something that they have invested in, and we do suggest that the Sunday cook-a-thon include them as soon as they can hold a knife—whether you're making the Bonus Week meals or any others. You can start them around age two with a plastic "lettuce knife" and let them cut up salad greens, then graduate to a serrated bread knife, which is easier to handle and harder to cut oneself with. By age three, they can handle a small paring knife if watched and guided well. I have taught many six-, seven-, and eight-year-olds to use a ten-inch chef's knife safely as long as they are the kind of kid who can keep their eye on the job.

HOW TO USE THIS BOOK

EACH WEEK HAS a work schedule that outlines how you are going to accomplish a week's worth of healthy cooking in three or so hours. Getting everything prepared on Sunday so that cooking the evening meal on any day later in the week in a simple, one-step process is the foundation of this book. The work schedule will help you plan the preparations, and the end result on a busy weeknight will be almost like stopping for takeout on the way home and warming it up in your own oven. Except cheaper, healthier, and yummier!

Here's how to get going:

◆ When starting a meal plan, set out all recipe ingredients in groups around the kitchen. You don't need any special equipment or a large space by any means. The idea is that you use your space well: one side of the sink for veggies, one side for raw meat; one side of your stove for cooking one dish, and the other for cooking the second dish or prepping something else.

◆ The recipes are in order of what you start first so you can read each week's recipes from beginning to end and just keep moving until all of your ingredients are off the counter and in the pots. Once you get going, it will become clear what needs to happen next. For instance, when you hit a point in the first recipe that says "simmer for 20 minutes" you can move on to the next recipe and get it started. By having "stations" around the stove, you can see what goes where and you won't have to keep checking the recipe and running to the fridge. Your first attempt may be a bit clumsy, but don't give up! Like anything, the routine will become, well, routine. Each week is designed to ease you further into the process, starting with the simplest and moving to the more complex.

◆ A note about garbage: always keep a large bowl for discards in a convenient space on the counter when working. This eliminates the unnecessary steps to your garbage can or compost bin over and over again. Emptying one container at the end of the cooking session is much more hygienic and efficient than making several dozen trips to the trash. If you'd like, you can place one bowl next to your stove and one next to your sink directly in front of you.

◆ Assess your storage needs. If you want to store your soups in single-serving sizes because your family eats at different times, then please do so. If you are the set-the-casserole-on-the-table kind of household, then be sure to freeze it all in one container. The reheating instructions are intended to be flexible and you can adjust the reheating times up or down depending on your needs. It is always better to freeze in shallow containers because the freezing process happens more quickly, keeping food fresher, and the reheating process is faster.

As you go along, you will find that you always have one or two dishes in the freezer for quick meals. When you find that a dish is a hit with the whole family, be sure to double it next time you make it and freeze for future use.

We have provided you with grocery lists for each week. Each list has all of the ingredients that you need for that week. Once you are sure which meals will go over with everyone (and we have plenty of variation ideas for the fussiest members) you can photocopy the list to increase the amount of each ingredient as needed to double or triple a recipe. Or visit www.cookonceaweek.com. You will find all the shopping lists there for you in downloadable form.

When you have a complete list of all that you need for the weekly plan (including your up- or downsizing, if necessary), you can photocopy this plan multiple times so you can use it over again throughout the season. Try keeping a binder with these shopping lists and tracking your grocery bills. Family life being the circus that it is, we are sure the other copies will get misplaced, splattered upon, or chewed by the dog. Do yourself a favor and keep this copy. Don't lose sight of this page of crucial information!

At the end of each week there is a blank page, ready to be filled with your notes. What did your kids like best? Did you change up some spicing, increase serving sizes? Write it down so you won't forget.

All weeks are designed to cost approximately $85.00 for the foundation of the meals, assuming that you have a few of the staples on hand. Storage containers and sealable freezer bags will cost extra but can be reused often.

Good luck and enjoy all the free time that *Cook Once a Week, Eat Well Every Day* will give you!

GETTING ORGANIZED

ONE OF THE things I do in the coaching role of my job is to show people how to get through that planning, shopping, and cooking process more efficiently. I am amazed at how many people try to skip that step of planning. Then they are, in turn, amazed at how much food rots in their fridge. The process is detailed, but here are my best tips.

Shopping

- Find out which day your market gets produce deliveries and shop on those days. The best idea is to shop and cook on the same day so you can skip the step of putting things away!
- Always shop at the same store because you will get to know what they carry and where to find it quickly.
- Try to shop early in the day or later in the evening, when stores are quieter.
- Take your list with you. Do not try to "remember" at the store.
- When shopping, be sure to gather all items from the perimeter of the store first. Typically, fresh items will be found there, and you'll need only a very few minutes in specific aisles to gather canned or packaged goods.
- Take extra produce bags and use them for meat but skip them for most veggies because they are another unnecessary step.
- Using a bin or a box instead of grocery bags saves time at the store and at home, not to mention the environmental bonus. Just pack your own bins and put similar things in one bin—pantry items, fresh meat with dairy and vegetables, canned goods. When you get home, it will be easy to assign one person to the cupboard and one to the fridge for unpacking duties.
- Store ingredients when possible in their recipe grouping. Keeping all of the vegetables for a certain soup in one bag or corner makes a quicker start.
- If you are lucky enough to live in an urban center with online shopping and delivery, be sure to save your list in their system so you only have to shop once and your precious list will be there to use again.

Cooking

- Take out all required pots and bowls to start.
- Clean and chop all veggies for all recipes at once so you are not running from the sink to the stove.
- Fry all onions (or common ingredients such as celery, peppers, etc.) required in one pan, then separate them into pots as needed.
- Get one recipe under control or to the "simmer for . . ." stage before moving on to the next.

◆ If you modify a recipe, make notes so you will be able make the same changes each time.

Storing

◆ Choose shallow, long storage containers if possible. They will cool and freeze more efficiently, preserving vitamins and improving food safety; they will also thaw and reheat faster.

◆ Move a finished product from the hot to the cold stage as quickly as possible. Do not cool on the counter. It is safer to put items in the fridge away from such perishables as meat and milk.

◆ Label items with tape and a permanent marker and include the date. You might remember, but chances are you won't. I don't and I do this for a living. The time used solving mysteries from your freezer is better spent just about anywhere else.

A Bit about **BREAKFAST** and **LUNCH**

BREAKFAST

SOME OF THE most stressful moments in any family household are during the morning hours. Our picture of the 1950s mom in the kitchen calling the boys to a breakfast of bacon and eggs with toast and juice seems almost absurd in today's harried life. But there are ways to make breakfast go smoothly and to take the pressure off. A box of cereal is not really the answer as it provides mostly carbohydrates and very little protein. The grumbly tummy will be looking for more sugar by recess. A few hints on breakfast are all you need because it is the most often repeated meal of the week. You would not dream of serving the same pizza five days in a row, but often today's breakfast looks just like yesterday's.

The secret is in the planning. When you have time on the weekend to prepare a few things, why not make a few more and freeze them for the week?

Breakfast Plan 1: French Toast

French toast is a chameleon, with protein, omega-3 fatty acids, whole grains, calcium, and then some. It has many faces and is great to make ahead and freeze to be microwaved for one to two minutes on high during the weekday rush.

Basic French Toast: Stir together 1 egg, 2 tablespoons milk, ½ teaspoon sugar, and ½ teaspoon cinnamon for each slice of whole wheat bread. Scale up per person, each adult will need two slices, each child under eight will need one per meal. (Add extra bread for cooking now to freeze for the week.) Soak bread in the egg mixture for a few minutes. Fry in a nonstick pan sprayed with cooking spray over medium heat until brown; flip and brown the other side (about 2 minutes per side). Eat now, or wrap in foil and freeze in a zip-top bag.

Variations

Buttermilk French Toast: Use low-fat buttermilk instead of milk for a creamier texture. The nutrients are the same but the fluffier texture is sometimes more appealing.

Juicy French Toast: Substitute orange, apple, pineapple, or any favorite juice in place of the milk and omit the sugar in the main recipe.

English Muffin or Bagel French Toast: Substitute any type of bread for a change.

Shapes Toast: Allow kids to use cookie cutters to shape their toast any way they like. Try to use large cutters to reduce waste. Don't throw away the crusts: just eat them yourself.

Stuffed French Toast: Ham and cheese sandwiches can be turned into Croque Monsieurs by dipping in egg mixture and frying. Any of your favorite lunch fillings work.

Apple Cheesecake French Toast: Put cream cheese and apple slices between two pieces of hot, cooked French toast with a little sprinkle of cinnamon.

Toppings

Of course maple syrup is called for but you can reduce its use by providing other toppings. Fruit is always at the top of the list for adding vitamins and fiber into each meal.

Frozen Blueberry Compote: Bring 2 tablespoons each of water and granulated sugar to a boil and dissolve. Add 1 cup frozen blueberries and bring to a boil; lower heat and simmer for 5 minutes. Store in fridge up to 2 weeks.

Frozen Strawberry Compote: Bring 2 tablespoons each of water and sugar to a boil and dissolve. Add 1 cup frozen strawberries and bring to a boil; lower heat and simmer for 5 minutes. Store in fridge up to 2 weeks.

Apple Compote: This is great for those apples that are going a little soft. Keep the skins on if you can get away with it. Just scrub and rinse well and chop off bruised bits. Bring 2 tablespoons each of water and sugar to a boil and dissolve. Add 1 cup chopped apples and 1 teaspoon cinnamon and bring to a boil; lower heat and simmer for 5 minutes. Store in fridge up to 2 weeks.

Breakfast Plan 2: Muffins for Breakfast

One of the problems with breakfast is its reputation. It can be a boring meal that is pressure filled since it truly is the foundation of the day. Breaking fast is important for the growing (or groaning) brain that has used up all of its fuel overnight and just can't get into gear without something to burn. To take the pressure off, why not let breakfast seem like dessert? You can feel good about serving any one of our desserts for breakfast (see recipes on pages 159 to 174), because they are all designed with nutrition in mind and—while they have sugar—have healthy doses of protein, fruits, and vegetables. I suggest one of our muffin recipes. Sometimes getting vegetables into a child means hiding them, and that means baking. Sweet Potato Muffins (page 163) or Zucchini Muffins (page 164) are good disguises that contain a whole grain, some vegetables, and some protein from the eggs. Even one of these and a glass of milk is a balanced meal.

Breakfast Plan 3: Shake It Up

Think of your blender as your best friend. Let kids fill it the night before to refrigerate with any combination of the ingredients below. Pick one from each column and simply blend them together in the morning. Each pitcher will serve two to three people.

LIQUID	FRUIT	PROTEIN	ADD-INS
2 cups vanilla soymilk	1 banana	2 tablespoons almond butter	1 teaspoon ground flaxseed
2 cups chocolate soy milk	½ cup frozen raspberries	½ cup silken tofu	1 teaspoon cinnamon
2 cups milk	2 tablespoons frozen blueberries	1 teaspoon peanut butter	1 teaspoon vanilla extract
2 cups orange juice	½ cup applesauce		1 teaspoon wheat germ

Breakfast Plan 4: Whatever Works

There are a few of us who don't like breakfast at all and would prefer lunch food. Our culture is unique in its reliance on grains and specific breakfast meals. Many cultures simply have variations of the other meals in the morning hours. For instance, in Japan you would have rice, miso soup, and some kind of fish; in Mexico you would not be surprised to see beans on your plate. If your family has a favorite food, don't balk at reheating it for breakfast. It can be fun to have soup or chili at this meal once in a while. If they ask for it, break the rules and give it to them.

LUNCH

LUNCH STUMPS. IF you are forced to pack a lunch to send to school, then you have to walk the line between sending something familiar, so your kids don't get teased, and sending something nutritious. In most school lunchrooms, you will see more packaged foods than homemade lunches. You will also see the dessert eaten first, the fruit thrown into the garbage, and more talking than eating going on. If your children are sent to school with a good breakfast, you can breathe easily knowing that they will make it through the day without starving, so there is no need to go to the lowest common denominator to get them to "eat something, anything!" Liquid is most important here. A good drink will keep their bodies from becoming dehydrated and that is just as important as whatever solid is packed for lunch. The trick here, then, is a glass of milk (preferably purchased from school so you don't have to stock and transport it) and something interesting enough for them to nibble.

If milk is not available at school, then invest in a few small containers that you can pour milk into and partially freeze so it stays cold. (Nothing turns kids off milk faster than a big gulp of sour milk.) A tiny packet of chocolate powder is not the end of the world and it is a better option than buying the chocolate milk itself. Although I am dead against the caffeine in cocoa being fed to kids, some kids simply won't drink white milk, and at least you can control the amount by packaging a teaspoon of chocolate milk powder mixed with a teaspoon of instant dry powdered milk to boost the calcium. Letting the kids mix it themselves adds to the fun.

Veggie Strategies

The big hurdle is vegetables. Being realistic about what our kids will eat out of our sight means making the food as attractive as possible and keeping portions small. Do not send what you know they will waste. Letting them see your commitment to vegetables sets up a lifelong brainwashing, in a good way. Invest in a crinkle cutter so your carrot sticks look all wiggly and your celery stuffed with cream cheese has a wavy appearance. Dips are a good idea, too. Pick up some tiny containers that you can fill with salsa or guacamole at best or bottled dressing at worst. Hey, whatever gets it in. A few vegetables dipped into Very Cheesy Yogurt Dip (1 cup plain, low-fat yogurt mixed with ½ cup shredded Cheddar cheese and 1 teaspoon low-fat mayonnaise) and a handful of whole-grain, trans-fat-free crackers make for a decent lunch. For extra vegetables, take a look at our recipe for Krispy Kale (page 60). If it is packed in a hard container, it will travel well, and the similarity to potato chips makes it acceptable to younger tongues.

Meat and Other Proteins

Another thing that you want in that lunch box is some protein. Our kids, being the carbohydrate hounds that they are, most often prefer bread with something on it, but even they get bored of that, so try some of these ideas:

Meat "Fries": Slice a few pieces of meat from Sunday dinner into French-fry shapes and send some ketchup or mustard for them to dip.

Lunch Rolls: These are simply sliced meats rolled around a slice of apple or melon and stuck with a toothpick. Try prosciutto or turkey meat rather than ham or bologna. Prosciutto is dry cured without nitrites, and turkey is leaner than the other two.

Soups, Stews, Pasta: The Thermos needs to make a comeback. Send any of the soups or stews that the kids like from your supper meals. Pasta is great, too. Fresh spinach tortellini has fiber and folic acid in it and, if you buy the fresh product made with whole eggs, you are getting extra protein. It is a nice treat, especially if you send some tomato sauce as a dip.

Hot Dogs: These can go in a Thermos for a good surprise. Try veggie hot dogs early in life and the kids will like them more than the beef kind, but even chicken is a leaner choice than beef. Be sure to boil them beforehand and place in a Thermos to keep them at a safe temperature until lunch. Wrap favorite toppings in snack-size containers to go along with the bun.

Grab and Go Lunches: Many of our dinner meals have "Grab & Go Lunch" ideas that use, as their foundation, the cooked key ingredients from the previous meals. These tips offer ideas for what to include to create a wholesome lunch. For instance, one recipe calls for you to wrap last night's roasted chicken in a whole wheat tortilla with light mayonnaise, plain yogurt, and curry powder and send, along with crudités, for lunch. Wraps are great because they use much less bread to get the job done, and whole wheat or spinach wraps are more nutritious bite for bite than the plain variety. (Be sure to check the label because some wraps do contain partially hydrogenated shortening, which contains trans-fatty acids.)

Lunch-ables: There are some great containers that have little compartments so you can make your own lunch pack. How about a Make-Your-Own Pizza with mini whole wheat pitas in one compartment, tomato sauce in another, and shredded cheese in the third? A few slices of meat can go into another container, and the kids can build the pizza at school. Or try tuna in one section, whole-grain crackers in another, and baby carrots or cottage cheese, plus strawberries and a zucchini mini-muffin (page 164).

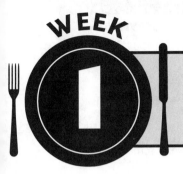

BASICS BUT BETTER

THIS MENU STARTS you off with a truly simple, no-fail week. These recipes are very familiar yet have simple adjustments to make them healthier and easier. The Better Spaghetti Sauce recipe is my secret weapon. Not a week goes by that I don't use some version of this, which is always in my freezer. Our family loves its sweetness, which is provided by the vegetables (but don't tell them that!). If I don't have ground beef, I use ground chicken. If I have vegetarians over, I use vegetarian ground meat substitute, which is textured vegetable protein (it is available at health food stores and in the prepared-foods aisle of many supermarkets). I serve it in every combination imaginable: over pasta, in wraps, as a pizza topping, or just out of the microwave, with a spoon (while I take a four-minute lunch break like every other mother I know).

I was demonstrating the flexibility of this recipe once on a television program while my husband and daughter watched from home—she was about eight years old. As I was grating onion and various other "gross" vegetables into the sauce, my husband had to hold back laughter while my daughter looked on in horror. "No way, she puts that in it? Ewwww, I am never eating spaghetti again!" she said. Her resolve only lasted a few hours when she figured out that it tasted good anyway.

WEEK 1 MENU CHART

SERVE	MAIN DISH	SERVE WITH
TONIGHT	Roasted Chicken to Please Everybody	No extras needed
2ND NIGHT	Better Spaghetti Sauce	Salad
3RD NIGHT	Pork Roast Dijon with Sweet Potatoes	Steamed Snow Peas
4TH NIGHT	Better Nachos	Carrots and celery sticks
5TH NIGHT	Baked Pork & Spinach Roll-Up	Cherry tomato salad
GRAB & GO LUNCH	Beef Burritos	
GRAB & GO LUNCH	Chicken Salad Wrap	
Grab & Go Lunch	Chop Suey Chicken Salad	

= Second Supper recipe

WORK SCHEDULE

1. Start spaghetti sauce first, as it needs to simmer while you prepare the remaining recipes. Half of this can be stored in the fridge to use this week and the other half should be frozen in single serving sizes for up to 4 weeks.

2. Prepare veggies for the chicken dish and lay on baking sheet.

3. Rinse chicken, pat dry with paper towel, and place in its roasting pan; cover with plastic wrap and refrigerate.

4. Prepare both pieces of pork and place in zip-top freezer bag in freezer.

5. Sweet potatoes can be stored in a cool dry cupboard and snow peas in the fridge for the night that you are serving Pork Roast Dijon.

6. Optional step: Prep, wash, and store carrot sticks and celery sticks to serve with Better Nachos.

7. Prepare snow peas only when you are ready to serve the Pork Roast Dijon dinner.

Better Spaghetti Sauce

SERVES: 4 as entrée + 4 for Second Supper + 1 to 2 for Grab & Go Lunch
PREPARATION TIME: 30 minutes

Cook this sauce *today and have options all week. This recipe rinses away much of the saturated fat and loads up on hidden vegetables, which virtually disappear during the cooking process. It contains four to five times as much vegetable as meat, a healthy ratio. Divide this sauce in half, serve half for tomorrow night's supper over about a pound of spinach pasta or whole wheat spaghetti, and store the balance in 2-cup containers until ready to use as Second Supper and / or Grab & Go Lunch.*

1 pound extra-lean ground beef
1 teaspoon canola oil
1 onion, grated
2 carrots, grated
1 green bell pepper, seeded, cored, and grated
3 cloves garlic, minced
1 tablespoon Italian herb seasoning
1 teaspoon fennel seed (optional)
2 cups frozen mashed winter squash (see Tips)
1 (26-ounce) can tomato sauce
1 (5½-ounce) can tomato paste
1 cup red wine
¼ cup ground flaxseed (see Tips)

◆ In skillet, brown meat over medium-high heat; place meat in a strainer in sink. Run under hot water to drain as much of the fat as possible. Set aside.

◆ In large saucepan, heat oil over medium-high heat; cook onion, carrots, and green pepper until softened. Add cooked ground beef. Stir in garlic and Italian seasoning. Add fennel seed (if using).

◆ Add squash and heat through. Add tomato sauce, tomato paste, and wine. Simmer for at least 20 minutes or for up to 1½ hours.

◆ Divide sauce into two portions. Store half in fridge for tomorrow night's supper, freeze second half in 2-cup portions for use in Better Nachos (page 16).

◆ Stir ground flaxseed into sauce only after sauce has been rewarmed for eating, to preserve all of the seeds' nutrients; omega-3 fatty acids in flax can be degraded very quickly if heated.

TIPS

THE GROUND FLAXSEED is stirred into the sauce at the end of cooking to maintain all of its "good fats." This invisible seed adds fiber. Do not use the seed whole because our bodies cannot break down the hull to digest all of the goodness.

Frozen mashed squash is not always available but canned pumpkin or cubed fresh or frozen squash is a good substitute. Simply add it and mash with a fork as it cooks and softens.

Better Nachos

These nachos are a delicious and balanced meal when served with salsa and carrot and celery sticks.

> 2 to 4 cups Better Spaghetti Sauce
> 1 (14-ounce) package low-salt corn chips
> 1 to 2 cups shredded Cheddar cheese
> 1 cup salsa
> Carrot and celery sticks, for serving

REHEAT ONE OF the leftover Better Spaghetti Sauce servings in microwave. Empty the package of low-salt corn chips onto a platter, top with warmed sauce then shredded Cheddar cheese. Broil for 1 to 2 minutes to melt cheese. Top with salsa and serve.

SERVES: 4 ➤ PREPARATION TIME: 5 minutes

Beef Burritos

IF THERE IS any sauce left over, wrap in whole wheat tortillas and then individually in plastic wrap. These are great for lunch microwaved for 1 to 2 minutes per wrap and served with an apple.

SERVES: 1 to 2 ➤ PREPARATION TIME: 1 minute

COOK ONCE A WEEK, EAT WELL EVERY DAY

Roasted Chicken to Please Everybody

> **SERVES:** 4 as entrée + 2 for Grab & Go Lunch
> **PREPARATION TIME:** 15 minutes

This is a *versatile recipe that allows everyone—kids and adults—to get what they want by removing the kids' portions before the extra garlic and herb flavorings are added. Ask the butcher (even at the grocery store) to remove the backbone of the chicken, which reduces the cooking time by eliminating the need to heat the empty chicken cavity. To remove the backbone yourself, grip the tail with a paper towel and hold firmly while you slide a sharp knife up the back along one side of the spine, cutting away from you. You will reach some resistance when you get to the middle back but holding the bird upside down and pushing your knife downward toward the cutting board will give you the leverage needed.*

2 red potatoes
3 carrots
1 small rutabaga
1 onion
2 tablespoons garlic oil or any other flavored oil
1 chicken (3 to 4 pounds), backbone removed
1 head garlic
¼ cup white wine (see Tips)
Salt and pepper to taste
1 sprig fresh tarragon

◆ Wash and scrub potatoes and carrots but do not peel; roughly chop into 2-inch pieces. Peel and roughly cube rutabaga into 1-inch pieces. Quarter onion, then peel and discard skin.
◆ Spread the vegetables on foil-lined baking sheet; drizzle with half of the garlic oil.
◆ Rinse chicken under cold running water; pat dry with paper towel. Place in shallow roasting pan, skin side up. Break head of garlic in half; place unpeeled under chicken. Press down on chicken to flatten slightly. Mix wine, remaining oil, salt and pepper; drizzle over chicken. At this point you may cover with plastic wrap and refrigerate for up to 24 hours.
◆ To cook, preheat oven to 350°F. Roast chicken and vegetables in 350°F oven for 1½ hours or until meat thermometer registers 185°F and juices run clear when chicken is pierced. The vegetables should be tender.

- Carve and remove pieces the children prefer. Return to roasting pan remaining portions for adults.
- Preheat broiler. Remove garlic halves and squeeze the flesh from the papery skins into a bowl. Coarsely chop tarragon leaves and mix into garlic. If desired, remove as much chicken skin as possible to reduce calories and fat. Using fork, smear garlic paste onto chicken pieces reserved for adults. Broil for 2 minutes. Serve with roasted vegetables.

TIPS

REMOVE ALL LEFTOVER meat from bones and store in fridge up to 3 days to use for Grab & Go Lunch or freeze up to 3 weeks. The chicken carcass can be broken and boiled in 6 cups water with 1 chopped yellow or Spanish onion (with the skin on, for color) to make stock or to be frozen for 3 weeks.

If you won't drink the remaining wine in the bottle, search for mini bottles. Many retailers carry a 300mL size that will do for just a recipe or two. You could also use other alcohol here—the sherry left over from Christmas, the beer in the fridge, the grappa from that Mediterranean party. Chicken stock is always a good substitute if you are avoiding alcohol.

Chicken Salad Wrap

CHOP REMAINING CHICKEN and mix with 1 tablespoon each plain yogurt and mayonnaise, just enough to moisten, as well as 1 teaspoon curry powder. Use the chicken salad to fill whole wheat wraps. Eat within three days. Pack any crudités you have to round out the lunch.

SERVES: 1 to 2 ➤ **PREPARATION TIME:** 2 minutes

Chop Suey Chicken Salad

LEFTOVER CHICKEN CAN be chopped along with cooked root vegetables from the night before and tossed with 2 tablespoons low-sodium soy sauce, 1 teaspoon Dijon mustard, and ½ teaspoon toasted sesame oil. Serve on mixed greens for a great lunch salad. A few rice crackers can be crushed and sprinkled on top for low-fat croutons.

SERVES: 1 to 2 ➤ **PREPARATION TIME:** 2 minutes

Pork Roast Dijon with Sweet Potatoes

SERVES: 4 as entrée + 4 for Second Supper
PREPARATION TIME: 10 minutes

This roast is *wonderful served with Steamed Snow Peas (recipe follows).*

²⁄₃ cup ground almonds (see Tip)
2 cups white wine
6 tablespoons Dijon mustard
1 teaspoon pepper
Two (2-pound) rolled boneless pork center loin roasts
4 small sweet potatoes, scrubbed
1 teaspoon olive oil
Salt and pepper to taste

◆ In large zip-top plastic bag, combine almonds, wine, mustard, and pepper. Add roasts and smear almond mixture all over meat. (Seal bag and refrigerate for up to 3 days. Or freeze for up to 3 weeks; thaw in refrigerator for 24 to 48 hours.)

◆ Cut sweet potatoes into eight wedges each. Place in large zip-top plastic bag along with oil, salt, and pepper; shake to coat. (Refrigerate for up to 48 hours.)

◆ Preheat oven to 375°F. Arrange potatoes in single layer on foil-covered baking sheet. Place both roasts fat side up, and as much almond mixture as possible, in shallow roasting pan. Roast potatoes on upper rack and pork on lower rack of 375°F oven for 60 to 90 minutes, or until meat thermometer reaches 160°F, adding ¼ cup more wine if pan starts to burn.

◆ Let roast sit for 5 minutes or so to allow juices to settle, then carve. While carving the roast, be sure to cube the second roast into 1-inch pieces before storing. This way, your Second Supper is in the bag!

TIP

GROUND ALMONDS BOOST the protein and good fat. They can be found in the baking section of the grocery store.

Steamed Snow Peas

SERVES: 4
PREPARATION TIME: 3 minutes

2 cups fresh snow pea pods
1 tablespoon white wine or lemon juice
1 teaspoon granulated sugar
Salt and pepper to taste

◆ Rinse snow peas under cold water and place in large microwavable bowl; sprinkle with wine, sugar, salt, and pepper. (Can be covered with plastic wrap and refrigerated up to 24 hours.)
◆ Microwave, covered, on high for 2 to 4 minutes, or until bright green and crisp-tender.
◆ To prepare in a steamer: steam washed snow peas for 2 to 4 minutes, toss with wine, sugar, salt, and pepper.

Baked Pork and Spinach Roll-Ups

2 pounds cooked Pork Roast Dijon, cubed
2 cups low-fat grated Cheddar cheese
1 (10-ounce) package prewashed baby spinach
8 whole wheat flour tortillas
Cooking spray
2 pints cherry tomatoes
2 teaspoons store-bought balsamic vinaigrette

◆ Toss chopped pork roast with Cheddar cheese and baby spinach leaves.
◆ Divide the mixture between the whole wheat tortillas and wrap up the filling burrito style. Lay the roll-ups in a single layer in a large casserole dish that has been coated with cooking spray.
◆ Preheat oven to 400°F. Bake uncovered at 400°F for 15 to 20 minutes just to warm through and melt cheese.
◆ Serve with a side salad of cherry tomatoes that have been halved and tossed with your favorite balsamic vinaigrette.

SERVES: 4 ➤ **PREPARATION TIME:** 5 minutes

YOU NEED:

Baked goods:
- ◯ 🥣 Whole wheat tortillas (16)

Dairy:
- ◯ 🥣 Cheddar cheese, shredded (3 to 4 cups)
- ◯ 🥣 Plain yogurt (1 tablespoon)

Meat and Alternatives:
- ◯ Extra-lean ground beef or veggie substitute (1 pound)
- ◯ Chicken (3 to 4 pounds), backbone removed
- ◯ Rolled boneless pork roast (two 2-pound)

Produce:
- ◯ Red potatoes (2)
- ◯ Green bell pepper (1)
- ◯ Sweet potatoes (4 small)
- ◯ Rutabaga (1 small)
- ◯ Fresh tarragon (1 sprig)
- ◯ Garlic (2 heads)
- ◯ Snow pea pods (2 cups)
- ◯ Carrots (7 to 9)
- ◯ Lemon juice (1 teaspoon) (optional)
- ◯ Onions (2)
- ◯ 🥣 Baby spinach (10-ounce package)
- ◯ 🥣 Celery (1 head) for crudités
- ◯ 🥣 Cherry tomatoes (2 pints)
- ◯ 🥣 Mixed greens (10-ounce package)
- ◯ 🥣 Apples (1 or 2)

Frozen Foods:
- ◯ Frozen mashed winter squash (16-ounce package)

CHECK YOUR PANTRY FOR:

Condiments and Dressings:
- ◯ Dijon mustard (6 tablespoons)
- ◯ 🥣 Balsamic vinaigrette (2 teaspoons)
- ◯ 🥣 Light mayonnaise (1 tablespoon)
- ◯ 🥣 Low-sodium soy sauce (2 tablespoons)

Cooking Oils:
- ◯ Garlic oil or other flavored oil (2 tablespoons)
- ◯ Canola oil (1 teaspoon)
- ◯ Olive oil (1 teaspoon)
- ◯ 🥣 Toasted sesame oil ($^{1}/_{2}$ teaspoon)

Pastas and Tomato Products
- ◯ Spinach pasta or whole wheat spaghetti (1 pound)
- ◯ Tomato paste ($5^{1}/_{2}$-ounce can)
- ◯ Tomato sauce (26-ounce can)
- ◯ Salsa (8 ounces)

Baking Products:
- ◯ Ground almonds ($^{2}/_{3}$ cup)
- ◯ Granulated sugar (1 teaspoon)

Spices and Seasonings:
- ◯ Fennel seed (1 teaspoon) (optional)
- ◯ Italian herb seasoning (1 tablespoon)
- ◯ 🥣 Curry powder (1 teaspoon)

Snack Foods:
- ◯ 🥣 Low-salt corn chips (14-ounce package)
- ◯ 🥣 Rice crackers (3 to 4 ounce package)

Health Foods:
- ◯ Ground flaxseed ($^{1}/_{4}$ cup)

Wine and Beer:
- ◯ Red wine (1 cup)
- ◯ White wine ($2^{1}/_{4}$ cups plus 1 tablespoon)

KEY: 🥣 denotes Second Supper or Grab & Go Lunch items

SHOPPING LIST

Notes:

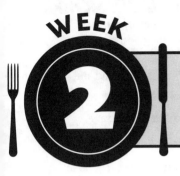

ENTERTAINING THE WHOLE FAM DAMILY

FROM TIME TO time in our neighborhood, usually right around dinnertime, come the jingly tinkles of the ice-cream truck. Once I overheard a slightly exasperated father calmly tell his three-year-old, "Yes, son, that is the vegetable truck." While my husband and I chuckled at his ingenuity at first, some uneasiness about this approach later set in. What worries me is the unspoken lesson: vegetables are yucky and you wouldn't want them. Kids these days, we are told, are overwhelmed with stress and eat more bad food much earlier than we ever did. They therefore need the superhero powers that only vegetables can give them. We are doing them a huge favor when we expose them to as many vegetables as possible. Don't give up. Try raw, cooked, and even frozen. Why can't frozen broccoli be a "tree Popsicle"? Whatever works! Kids need to see a new food many times before they will try it, and making vegetables a positive part of their lives is a good first step.

WEEK 2 MENU CHART

SERVE	MAIN DISH	SERVE WITH
TONIGHT	Sunday Ham with Baked Potatoes	Veggie Platter
2ND NIGHT	Roasted Vegetable Soup	Whole-grain bread and Cheddar cheese
3RD NIGHT	Black Bean Nachos	No extras necessary
4TH NIGHT	Sunday Ham Reprise	Frozen green beans
5TH NIGHT	Roasted Vegetable Frittata	Crusty whole-grain bread and mixed greens
GRAB & GO LUNCH	Stuffed Mini Pitas	

 = Second Supper recipe

WORK SCHEDULE

1 Start roasted veggies for soup. When done, pull out 4 cups of veggies—2 cups to serve as a side dish for tonight's dinner as well as 2 cups to refrigerate for Second Supper Roasted Vegetable Frittata. Complete soup for freezing.

2 Complete Black Bean Nachos to freeze.

3 Prepare ham and scrub potatoes. Set in fridge until ready to cook for tonight's supper.

4 Chop veggies for platter to serve as an appetizer today, or store in fridge in zip-top plastic bag with a piece of paper towel and they will last at least 3 days to give you a head start for the week.

COOK ONCE A WEEK, EAT WELL EVERY DAY

Roasted Vegetable Soup

SERVES: 4 as entrée + 4 as a side dish with Sunday Ham + 4 for use in
Second Supper, Roasted Veggie Frittata
PREPARATION TIME: 20 minutes

Top this soup *with grated Parmesan and serve with whole-grain bread and Cheddar cheese on the side.*

1 head garlic
10 plum tomatoes
4 zucchini
3 red bell peppers
2 green bell peppers
1 sweet onion
3 cups frozen corn niblets
10 cups chicken stock (preferably homemade or frozen) (see Tips)
2 tablespoons store-bought pesto sauce (see Tips)
¼ cup grated Parmesan cheese (optional)

◆ Set oven to broil.
◆ Wrap garlic in foil.
◆ Slice tomatoes into ½-inch-thick rings. Chop zucchini and red and green peppers into bite-size pieces. Place foil-wrapped garlic in oven. Spread tomatoes, zucchini, and peppers on foil-covered baking sheets and broil, in batches and stirring halfway through, 4 inches from heat until starting to brown, 15 to 20 minutes.
◆ Coarsely chop onion; spread with corn on separate baking sheet. When zucchini mixture is cooked, remove it from the broiler and replace with the corn mixture. Broil for 10 to 15 minutes until niblets are brown, watching carefully to prevent burning.
◆ Leaving the wrapped garlic in the oven, remove corn mixture from broiler. Arrange 2 to 3 cups of the assorted veggies on platter for tonight; cover and refrigerate until ready to serve with ham.
◆ In large pot, bring stock to a simmer. Add remaining broiled vegetables and pesto sauce; cook for 5 minutes on low heat. Let cool. Turn off broiler but leave garlic in oven until softened; squeeze the roasted garlic into soup, top with Parmesan if desired.
◆ Freeze in single or multiple portions up to 4 weeks; to reheat, warm on stovetop in pot, stirring gently, or microwave for 2 to 10 minutes.

Roasted Veggie Frittata

Use the reserved veggies from Roasted Vegetable Soup to toss into this weeknight frittata.

8 eggs
¼ cup milk
1 tablespoon canola oil
2 cups reserved roasted veggies
2 tablespoons grated Parmesan cheese
1 loaf crusty whole-grain bread
1 (10-ounce) package prewashed mixed greens

◆ With a fork, mix together the eggs with the milk. Preheat oven to 450°F. In a cast-iron skillet (or nonstick skillet with a heat-resistant handle), heat the canola oil over medium-high heat; add eggs and cook for 2 minutes until they start to bubble. Add roasted vegetables and Parmesan cheese; place cast-iron or other oven-safe skillet into oven, uncovered, until heated through, 8 to 10 minutes. Serve with crusty whole-grain bread and a salad of mixed greens.

SERVES: 4 ➤ **PREPARATION TIME:** 12 minutes

Black Bean Nachos

SERVES: 4 as entrée + 3 for Grab & Go Lunch
PREPARATION TIME: 15 minutes

Here's a fast, *colorful meal for a busy weeknight. To keep calories and fat low, limit cheese and corn chips, or choose low-fat options.*

½ sweet onion, chopped
1 tablespoon olive oil
1 cup canned tomatoes, chopped
1½ cups frozen corn niblets
1 (19-ounce) can black beans, drained and rinsed
2 tablespoons lime juice
1 tablespoon chile powder
1 teaspoon dried oregano
8 ounces Cheddar cheese, shredded
1 (10-ounce) package frozen chopped spinach, thawed and squeezed dry
2 cups store-bought salsa
1 (12-ounce) package low-fat tortilla chips (see Tip)

◆ In saucepan, sauté onion in oil for about 8 minutes over medium-high heat, covered, until very soft. Stir in tomatoes, corn, black beans, lime juice, chile powder, and oregano; cook 5 minutes to heat through.

◆ Spoon into 8-inch casserole dish; sprinkle with half of the Cheddar. Arrange spinach over top. Spoon on half of the salsa. (Can be covered and refrigerated for up to 3 days or frozen for 4 weeks.)

◆ Preheat oven to 350°F. Bake, 20 to 25 minutes. Or, if directly from the freezer, in 350°F oven for 45 minutes. Arrange tortilla chips on ovenproof platter. Invert black bean mixture over chips; top with remaining Cheddar. Bake for 10 minutes. Serve with remaining salsa.

TIP

KEEP SOME CHIPS aside so the kids can have salsa, chips, and cheese for dinner if they are not keen on beans. Baby carrots and celery for dipping are all you need to balance this meal.

Stuffed Mini Pitas

CUT A SLIT in the tops of 9 mini whole wheat pitas and stuff leftovers, chips and all, into pitas. Place 3 stuffed pitas in each of three zip-top plastic bags and refrigerate up to 3 days. To serve, warm on plate in microwave for 1 minute. (Or place in a casserole dish in preheated oven at 400°F for 15 minutes.) Top with Cheddar cheese and reheat to melt it. Serve with chunks of avocado and a mini dish of salsa.

Serves: 1 to 2 ➤ PREPARATION TIME: 2 minutes

Sunday Ham with Baked Potatoes

SERVES: 4 as entrée + 4 for Second Supper
PREPARATION TIME: 20 minutes

Serve tonight with *a side dish of roasted veggies borrowed from the roasted vegetable soup (see page 25). Drizzle the vegetables with a little balsamic vinegar and olive oil.*

> 3 tablespoons whole cloves (see Tips)
> 1 (9-pound) cooked bone-in ham (see Tips)
> ¼ cup warm water
> ¼ cup honey mustard
> ¼ cup balsamic vinegar
> ¼ cup brown sugar
> 4 russet potatoes

- ◆ Preheat oven to 300°F.
- ◆ Poke cloves into ham in random pattern. Place ham in roasting pan. Mix warm water, mustard, vinegar, and brown sugar; pour over ham. Scrub potatoes; poke a few holes to let steam escape so they don't burst.
- ◆ Bake ham in its dish, and potatoes directly on the rack, for up to 3 hours or until hot throughout and potatoes are tender. Slice the ham and wrap a portion, with some pan juices, in foil and a zip-top freezer bag to be refrigerated or frozen (up to 3 weeks) for Sunday Ham Reprise (see page 29). Serve the remaining portion with the remaining pan juices alongside the potatoes.

WHOLE CLOVES MAKE great potpourri. When your house is a little stuffy from a combination of dogs and kids, put a pot on the stove containing 2 cups water, ¼ cup vinegar, and a handful of cloves. Simmer for 10 to 60 minutes and your home will smell great. Just watch that the pot does not boil dry: add more water as needed.

Freeze the ham bone and any scraps for Sunday Ham Soup (page 59).

Remember that the ham is fully cooked and you are just heating through as well as flavoring the meat, so if you'd like you can reduce the temperature and increase the cooking time, or alternatively increase the temperature up to 400°F and reduce time to 1 hour, if either is more convenient. Whatever fits into your day better is the option to choose.

Sunday Ham Reprise

Reserved slices of Sunday Ham and pan juices
4 small sweet potatoes
3 cups frozen green beans
1 teaspoon butter or nonhydrogenated margarine

◆ Preheat oven to 375°F.
◆ Place the slices of Sunday Ham, still in their foil packets, on a baking sheet.
◆ Scrub and dry the sweet potatoes and place directly on the oven rack. Cook for 45 minutes or until tender. Remove the ham from the oven along with the potatoes.
◆ Microwave or steam green beans and top with teaspoon of butter or nonhydrogenated margarine just minutes before you are ready to serve.

SERVES: 4 ➤ **PREPARATION TIME:** 3 minutes

Veggie Platter

SERVES: 4
PREPARATION TIME: 20 minutes

*A*lways put out *a platter of veggies after school or just before supper. This is when kids are at their hungriest and are more likely to munch. Add some fruit once in a while and try fresh herbs; kids who won't touch salad might nibble on parsley or mint.*

> 2 bell peppers, one red, one yellow
> 1 head broccoli
> 1 head celery
> 2 cups fresh snow pea pods

◆ Rinse and dry all vegetables. Seed, core, and slice red and yellow peppers. Cut broccoli into florets. Cut broccoli stalks and celery into short lengths. Place in a zip-top plastic bag in fridge along with snow peas. Add paper towel to bag to wick away moisture, replacing when wet.

YOU NEED:

Baked Goods:
- ⬤ Whole-grain bread (1 large loaf plus 1 loaf)

Dairy:
- ○ Parmesan cheese, grated ($\frac{1}{4}$ cup + 2 tablespoons) (optional)
- ○ Cheddar cheese (1 pound)
- ○ ⬤ Butter or nonhydrogenated margarine (1 teaspoon)
- ○ ⬤ Eggs (8)
- ○ ⬤ Milk ($\frac{1}{4}$ cup)

Meat and Alternatives:
- ○ Ham, cooked bone in (9-pound)

Produce:
- ○ Plum tomatoes (10)
- ○ Red bell peppers (4)
- ○ Green bell peppers (2)
- ○ Yellow bell pepper (1)
- ○ Zucchini (4)
- ○ Russet potatoes (4)
- ○ Sweet onions (2)
- ○ Garlic (1 head)
- ○ Celery (1 head)
- ○ Broccoli (1 head)
- ○ Snow peas (2 cups)
- ○ Lime (1) or lime juice (2 tablespoons)
- ○ ⬤ Avocado (1)
- ○ ⬤ Mixed greens (10-ounce package)
- ○ ⬤ Baby Carrots (1 pound)
- ○ ⬤ Sweet potatoes (4)

Frozen Foods:
- ○ Frozen corn niblets ($4\frac{1}{2}$ cups)
- ○ Frozen chopped spinach (10-ounce package)
- ○ ⬤ Frozen green beans (3 cups)
- ○ Chicken stock (10 cups)

CHECK YOUR PANTRY FOR:

Condiments and Dressings
- ○ Honey mustard ($\frac{1}{4}$ cup)
- ○ Pesto sauce (2 tablespoons)
- ○ Salsa (16-ounce jar plus 2 ounces)
- ○ Balsamic vinegar ($\frac{1}{4}$ cup)

Cooking Oils
- ○ Olive oil (1 tablespoon)
- ○ ⬤ Canola oil (1 tablespoon)

Pastas and Tomato Products
- ○ Canned tomatoes (1 cup)

Canned Beans and Soup Broths:
- ○ Black beans (19-ounce can)

Baking Products:
- ○ Brown sugar ($\frac{1}{4}$ cup)

Spices and Seasonings:
- ○ Dried oregano (1 teaspoon)
- ○ Chile powder (1 tablespoon)
- ○ Whole cloves (3 tablespoons)

Snack Foods:
- ○ Low-fat tortilla chips (10-ounce package)

KEY: ⬤ denotes Second Supper or Grab & Go Lunch items

SHOPPING LIST

Notes:

COOK ONCE A WEEK, EAT WELL EVERY DAY

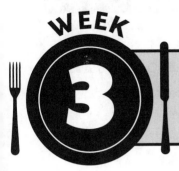

STANDARDS FACE-LIFT

WHILE WRITING THIS cookbook, I had many clients, friends, and colleagues offer to test my recipes and weekly plans. Although the individual recipes and meal plans work well for me when I'm cooking for clients, I wanted to be sure that the plans work for the "mom on the street." I outlined very loosely what I needed in terms of feedback but was more interested in seeing what mattered most to each tester. Some commented on the process, some were helpful about the taste and texture of each dish, and others paid special attention to the leftovers or shopping lists.

This week was tested by a biology professor, Julie Dais, who is a working mom with two kids. All of the above mattered to her, and her comments and suggestions were detailed and precise. I sat a little straighter in my chair when her feedback came in, as you would when your favorite teacher read your first draft. Other testers were perhaps a little easier on me, but their efforts were no less valuable. Learning what "mom on the street" wants from this book has given me a wealth of understanding and I thank all of my testers. So will you!

WEEK 3 MENU CHART

SERVE	MAIN DISH	SERVE WITH
TONIGHT	Pork Tenderloin with Spinach and Blue Cheese	Roasted Vegetables with Garlic Oil, Tomato Salad
2ND NIGHT	Chicken Cacciatore Stew in Pumpernickel Bowls	No extras necessary
3RD NIGHT	Salmon Cakes with Caper Mayo	Crudités
4TH NIGHT	🥣 Garlicky Roasted Vegetable Penne	Baby Spinach with Italian Dressing
5TH NIGHT	🥣 Spinach Linguine with Chicken Ragout	Mixed green salad
GRAB & GO LUNCH	Spinach and Blue Cheese Lunch Wrap	
GRAB & GO LUNCH	Pork and Cabbage Stir-Fry	

🥣 = Second Supper recipe

WORK SCHEDULE

1 Clean, chop, and bake vegetables for Roasted Vegetables with Garlic Oil.

2 Complete Chicken Cacciatore recipe up to simmer, then start on salmon.

3 Microwave or steam salmon for Salmon Cakes, then let cool while you make Caper Mayo and divide for Salmon Cakes as well as dip.

4 Continue with salmon recipe up to cornmeal step. Freeze for later in the week.

5 Start pork tenderloin recipe and store in fridge until ready to cook for tonight's supper. Continue with Tomato Salad. Cover and refrigerate.

6 Complete Chicken Cacciatore Stew and freeze for later in the week.

7 Get a head start on the week by cutting up any remaining vegetables for Crudités for Salmon Cakes night (optional).

Roasted Vegetables with Garlic Oil

> **SERVES :** 4 as entrée + 4 for Second Supper
> **PREPARATION TIME:** 20 minutes

The beautiful part *of this recipe is how un-needy it is. It cooks in about 30 minutes but can be left for up to 1 ½ hours in the oven and you don't have to worry about it a bit.*

1 large eggplant
4 small zucchini
3 medium-size red bell peppers
8 plum tomatoes
1 small onion
2 tablespoons garlic oil (see Tips)
Salt and pepper to taste
¼ cup dry Italian-seasoned bread crumbs
1 tablespoon dried basil

◆ Preheat oven to 350°F. Cut eggplant into chunks about one-quarter of the size of your palm and about ½ inch thick. Cut zucchini in half lengthwise. Seed, core, and cut bell peppers in half lengthwise; cut in half again. Halve tomatoes. Slice onion into rings.

◆ Brush large roasting pan or two baking dishes with half of the garlic oil. Arrange vegetables in one layer in pan; brush with remaining garlic oil. Sprinkle with salt and pepper. Bake until tender, stirring once or twice, about 30 minutes (or up to 1 ½ hours).

◆ Remove to serving platter. Sprinkle with bread crumbs and basil. Cover lightly with plastic wrap and let stand for up to 2 hours. Serve at room temperature, or broil for 3 minutes to reheat and crisp up the topping.

◆ Store leftovers (approximately 2 to 3 cups) in fridge covered with ⅛ cup extra-virgin olive oil and 2 tablespoons of balsamic vinegar to go into Second Supper, Roasted Vegetable Pasta. Refrigerate in airtight container for up to 4 days.

TIPS

IF GARLIC OIL is hard to find, try any seasoned oil. Or make your own by squeezing 2 cloves of garlic into 1 cup olive oil. Use what you need here and store the rest in the fridge for up to 4 weeks. For a quick way to make garlic bread, spread with seasoned oil and broil.

Garlicky Roasted Vegetable Penne

1 pound whole wheat penne or other small pasta
1 (19-ounce) can lupini or fava beans
1 clove garlic, crushed
2 to 4 cups reserved roasted vegetables
1 bunch fresh basil, chopped
2 tablespoons grated Parmesan cheese (optional)
1 (10-ounce) package prewashed baby or leaf spinach
Italian Dressing (page 178) or your favorite homemade or bottled dressing

BOIL WATER IN a large pot and add pasta. In a large microwavable bowl mix beans, undrained, with crushed garlic. Toss in reserved veggies with liquid and microwave at high for 3 to 5 minutes. When pasta is cooked, toss with vegetables in bowl. Chopped fresh basil and grated Parmesan cheese are welcome toppings. Serve with a spinach salad tossed with our Italian Dressing or your favorite dressing.

SERVES: 4 ➤ **PREPARATION TIME:** 8 minutes

Chicken Cacciatore Stew
in Pumpernickel Bowls

SERVES: 4 as entrée + 4 for Second Supper
PREPARATION TIME: 12 minutes

Some kids don't *like things all cooked together so when preparing this dish I often cook a few pieces of chicken thoroughly in the first step and keep them separate, then serve them with the sauce as a dip.*

2 pounds boneless skinless chicken thighs (see Tips)
2 teaspoons canola oil
1 onion, cut into rings
1 green bell pepper, cored, seeded, and chopped
6 cloves garlic
2 (24-ounce) cans tomato sauce
2 teaspoons dried oregano
2 teaspoons dried basil
1 teaspoon dried rosemary
$\frac{1}{2}$ teaspoon dried thyme
$\frac{1}{2}$ teaspoon hot pepper flakes
$\frac{1}{4}$ teaspoon ground black pepper
2 dashes Tabasco sauce
8 ounces mushrooms, sliced (optional)
1 cup frozen green peas
$\frac{1}{4}$ cup fresh parsley, chopped (optional)
4 large pumpernickel buns

◆ Cut chicken into pieces one-quarter the size of your palm. Heat a large, deep pot over medium-high heat, then pour in oil. Add chicken in two batches; just to brown on all sides, letting pan reheat before adding second batch. Remove from pan and set aside.

◆ Add onion, green pepper, and garlic; turn heat down to medium and cook until onion is tender.

◆ Add tomato sauce, oregano, basil, rosemary, and thyme to pot. Return chicken to pot; simmer over medium-low heat, uncovered, for 45 minutes, stirring occasionally.

◆ Add red pepper flakes, ground black pepper, and Tabasco sauce.

- ◆ (Remove half of the contents to freezable containers to serve as pasta sauce with spinach linguini later in the week or up to 4 weeks.)
- ◆ Add mushrooms, if using, and green peas to remaining portion as well as parsley, if desired.
- ◆ Refrigerate this half to serve as stew for up to 3 days. Reheat in microwave or in saucepan until warmed through and serve in pumpernickel buns that have been hollowed out to use as edible bowls.

TIPS

I RECOMMEND RINSING the chicken under cold tap water and drying with a paper towel since the processing of chicken can leave its own residue. Be very careful to use a separate sink basin if you have two, and keep other foods away until you have cleaned up well.

Chicken thighs are much juicier and higher in iron than breasts, although they are higher in fat. We've reduced some of the fat here by using skinless thighs.

Second Supper

Spinach Linguine with Chicken Ragout

3 to 4 cups reserved Chicken Cacciatore
1 pound spinach linguine (see Tip)
¼ cup grated Parmesan cheese
1 (10-ounce package) prewashed mixed greens
Salad dressing

PREPARE LINGUINE ACCORDING to package directions while you reheat sauce in microwave or on the stovetop in a pot. Toss together and empty onto a large platter, top with Parmesan cheese, and serve family style. Serve with mixed greens tossed with salad dressing.

SERVES: 4 ➤ PREPARATION TIME: 8 minutes

TIP

IF YOUR FAMILY doesn't like spinach pasta, try spelt or whole wheat pasta, both of which are more nutritious than standard white pasta or the other colored pastas.

Salmon Cakes with Caper Mayo

SERVES: 4 as entrée + 4 for Grab & Go Lunch
PREPARATION TIME: 15 minutes

Salmon brings a *lot to the table nutritionally because it's rich in omega-3 fatty acids, but I think you'll serve these simply because they taste great. The color alone is appetizing, and the taste is a delicate balance of sweet and salty.*

2 pounds fresh salmon fillets
¼ cup lime or lemon juice
1 cup finely chopped green onion
1 cup finely chopped fresh cilantro or parsley
1 cup light mayonnaise
2 tablespoons Dijon mustard
1 teaspoon chile powder
2 tablespoons drained capers
1⅓ cups dry Italian-seasoned bread crumbs
½ cup cornmeal (see Tips)
2 tablespoons olive oil
2 teaspoons unsalted butter
1 (10-ounce) package prewashed mixed greens
1 bunch fresh mint (optional)

◆ Cut fish into a few pieces; place on microwavable plate. (If you don't have a microwave, simply heat 1 inch of water in a large, low pot with a lid and add salmon, cover, and steam for 6 to 10 minutes, until cooked through.) Cover with vented plastic wrap; microwave at high for 6 to 8 minutes until opaque. Scrape flesh from skin and crumble into bowl; drizzle with lime juice. Add green onion and cilantro; mix lightly with fork.

◆ In separate bowl, mix mayonnaise, mustard, and chile powder; add half to salmon and mix with fork. Add capers to remaining mayonnaise mixture for Caper Mayo; set aside.

◆ Mix bread crumbs into salmon mixture until it holds together, adding more bread crumbs, 1 tablespoon at a time, if necessary. Form into eight cakes, approximately 3 inches in diameter and ¾ inch thick. Roll in cornmeal to coat. Cover with plastic wrap and refrigerate for at least 30 minutes and up to 24 hours. (Cakes can be frozen, separated by plastic wrap, in airtight container.)

◆ In heavy skillet, heat oil and butter over medium-high heat; fry cakes until crisp and golden brown on bottom, 3 to 5 minutes. Turn carefully only once; brown other side. Cover and let warm through, 8 to 10 minutes. Serve with Caper Mayo and mixed greens.

◆ (Freeze unused cakes individually wrapped in plastic wrap, then placed in zip-top plastic bag for up to 2 weeks. Cook from frozen over medium to medium-low heat for 15 to 20 minutes to obtain a crispy cake, or microwave on a plate for 2 to 5 minutes each for a softer version.)

◆ For Grab & Go Lunch, simply take one or two salmon cakes for lunch straight out of the freezer; by lunchtime they will be thawed and ready to eat cold or warmed for 2 minutes in the microwave. Add ½ red bell pepper sliced, and a nectarine or other fruit, for a light but filling lunch.

TIPS

THESE CAKES ARE a good way to introduce fish to your kids. Feel free to serve on whole wheat buns with ketchup and mustard to present them like burgers if that is what it takes. Adults are typically satisfied with a couple of cakes and a salad.

Cornmeal makes great cornbread, but an even easier way to use it up is to make polenta. Boil 2 cups water and add ½ cup cornmeal; simmer and stir for 10 to 15 minutes until it becomes very gooey. Add 1 tablespoon butter and salt and pepper to taste for a whole-grain side dish. Any leftovers can be emptied into a cake pan, covered, and refrigerated overnight. You can cut into squares and fry them for breakfast.

Skip the green stuff for the kids if they turn green just thinking about it. I have introduced many kids to greens using fresh herbs, and mint is the best place to start. It is minty and cool and they are often thrilled at how much it tastes like their chewing gum! Slip them some fresh mint as a garnish to start; there is folic acid in it and they will eat it.

Pork Tenderloin with Spinach and Blue Cheese

SERVES: 4
PREPARATION TIME: 5 minutes

---

*T*he pork tenderloin dish *is baked in a casserole but its components remain separate, which is the best of both worlds—an easy method of producing a meal that most kids will eat.*

    2 (1-pound) pork tenderloins
    3 (10-ounce) packages frozen chopped spinach, thawed and drained (see Tips)
    ¼ cup red wine
    2 cloves garlic, minced
    2 tablespoons balsamic vinegar
    2 teaspoons dried oregano
    Salt and pepper to taste
    6 ounces blue cheese or cream cheese, crumbled (see Tips)

◆ Cut each pork tenderloin on diagonal into four equal portions. Spread spinach in shallow casserole dish large enough to hold pork without crowding dish. Nestle pork into spinach. Sprinkle with wine, garlic, vinegar, oregano, salt, and pepper. Crumble blue cheese on and around pork, leaving an area uncovered if blue cheese is not popular. Cover with foil and refrigerate for up to 24 hours, or freeze for up to 2 weeks.

◆ Preheat oven to 350°F. Place pork, covered, in oven and roast for 20 to 25 minutes, until meat thermometer registers 160°F and hint of pink remains in the center. Serve with Tomato Salad (page 42). (Pork can be sliced, wrapped in plastic wrap, and refrigerated for up to 3 days or frozen for up to 3 weeks.)

TIPS

FROZEN CHOPPED SPINACH is the bargain of the century, both nutritionally and financially. It is picked at its peak, cleaned (and we know what a pain that can be!), chopped, and frozen. It is the second healthiest vegetable in our food system (next to kale) and it usually costs less than $2.

Use cream cheese as a substitute for blue cheese for a milder dish.

If this recipe is a hit, next time double the ingredients and make two casseroles. The second can be frozen, wrapped in foil from the bottom up. Thaw in the fridge about 48 hours before roasting as directed.

Tomato Salad

> **SERVES:** 4 as side dish + 2 as side dish for Grab & Go Lunch
> **PREPARATION TIME:** 12 minutes

2 pints cherry tomatoes, halved
½ cup chopped fresh basil
2 cloves garlic, minced
Salt and pepper to taste

◆ In a medium-size bowl, toss cherry tomatoes with basil, garlic, salt and pepper. (Salad can be covered and refrigerated for up to 24 hours.)

Pork and Cabbage Stir-Fry

USE LEFTOVER SLICES of pork in a stir-fry. In large skillet, heat 1 tablespoon canola oil; add one 16-ounce package precut coleslaw. Toss with ¼ cup low-sodium soy sauce and 2 tablespoons honey. Stir in 1 to 2 tablespoons toasted sesame oil. Slice pork into thin strips; stir in to reheat. Cook some egg noodles on the side; they are faster than rice and contain some extra protein from the eggs. Serve the stir-fry over the noodles.

SERVES: 1 to 3 ➤ **PREPARATION TIME:** 10 minutes

Spinach and Blue Cheese Lunch Wrap

ANY EXTRA SPINACH with blue cheese is a great lunch if wrapped in a whole wheat tortilla with a few slices of smoked turkey or prosciutto. Warm in microwave for 1 minute before serving with some fruit alongside.

SERVES: 1 to 2 **PREPARATION TIME:** 3 minutes

YOU NEED:

Baked Goods:
- ◯ Italian-seasoned bread crumbs (1⅓ cups plus ¼ cup)
- ◯ 4 large pumpernickel buns
- ◯ 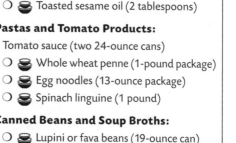 Whole wheat tortillas

Dairy:
- ◯ Blue cheese (6 ounces)
- ◯ Parmesan cheese, grated (¼ cup plus 2 tablespoons)
- ◯ Unsalted butter (2 teaspoons)

Meat and Alternatives:
- ◯ Fresh salmon fillets (2 pounds)
- ◯ Boneless skinless chicken thighs (2 pounds)
- ◯ Pork tenderloins (two 1-pound)
- ◯ Smoked turkey or prosciutto (6 slices)

Produce:
- ◯ Mixed greens (two 10-ounce packages)
- ◯ Green bell pepper (1)
- ◯ Plum tomatoes (8)
- ◯ Red bell peppers (4)
- ◯ Zucchini (4 small)
- ◯ Onions (2 small)
- ◯ Lime or lemon juice (¼ cup)
- ◯ Mushrooms, sliced (8 ounces) (optional)
- ◯ Green onions (1 bunch)
- ◯ Cherry tomatoes (2 pints)
- ◯ Fresh cilantro (1 bunch) (optional)
- ◯ Fresh mint (1 bunch) (optional)
- ◯ Fresh parsley (¼ cup) (optional)
- ◯ Eggplant (1 large)
- ◯ Garlic (11 cloves)
- ◯ Nectarines or other fruit (4)
- ◯ Coleslaw mix (16-ounce package)

Frozen Foods:
- ◯ Frozen chopped spinach (three 10-ounce packages)
- ◯ Frozen green peas (1 cup)

CHECK YOUR PANTRY FOR:

Condiments and Dressings
- ◯ Tabasco sauce (2 dashes)
- ◯ Dijon mustard (2 tablespoons)
- ◯ Capers (2 tablespoons)
- ◯ Light mayonnaise (1 cup)
- ◯ Balsamic vinegar (2 tablespoons)
- ◯ Low-sodium soy sauce (¼ cup)
- ◯ Honey (2 tablespoons)

Cooking Oils:
- ◯ Garlic oil (2 tablespoons)
- ◯ Canola oil (3 tablespoons)
- ◯ Olive oil (¼ cup plus 2 tablespoons)
- ◯ Toasted sesame oil (2 tablespoons)

Pastas and Tomato Products:
- Tomato sauce (two 24-ounce cans)
- ◯ Whole wheat penne (1-pound package)
- ◯ Egg noodles (13-ounce package)
- ◯ Spinach linguine (1 pound)

Canned Beans and Soup Broths:
- ◯ Lupini or fava beans (19-ounce can)

Baking Products:
- ◯ Cornmeal (½ cup)

Spices and Seasonings:

KEY: ⬤ denotes Second Supper or Grab & Go Lunch items

SHOPPING LIST

○ Chile powder (1 teaspoon)
○ Dried basil (5 teaspoons)
○ Hot pepper flakes ($\frac{1}{2}$ teaspoon)
○ Dried thyme ($\frac{1}{2}$ teaspoon)
○ Dried oregano (6 teaspoons)
○ Dried rosemary (1 teaspoon)

Wine and Beer:
○ Red wine ($\frac{1}{4}$ cup)

Notes:

KEY: 🥣 denotes Second Supper or
Grab & Go Lunch items

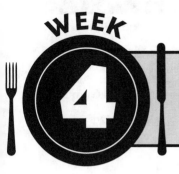

WEEK 4

WARMING FOOD FOR CHILLY DAYS

I AM LUCKY enough to have some of Toronto's best and brightest dieticians refer their clients to me. This happens when a client has learned that dietary improvements need to be made but needs help with the transition. With each referral, I learn a little more about specific dietary needs. One devoted health-care researcher and nutritional counsellor, Aileen Burford-Mason, is someone who can give you more information in five minutes than you could learn by yourself in a year. Her views are perhaps more "hard line" than mine, allowing no room for junk. I'm more "disguise and conquer." Aileen and I had a discussion about white rice that influenced this entire book.

I know that most of you are still eating white rice and I originally wrote most recipes for white rice (brown rice optional). Aileen encouraged me not to water down the message and to go the other way, using brown rice in recipes, making the white version the alternative. "If, and only if, it tastes better," I said. The result? You will find whole-grain brown rice in all of these recipes, and I encourage you to try them this way. They do taste better. Of course, nutritionally they really are better, whether you are counting carbs, vitamins and minerals, or fiber. Aileen and brown rice win.

WEEK 4 MENU CHART

SERVE	MAIN DISH	SERVE WITH
TONIGHT	Jamaican-ish Pork	Prepared Bean Salad with Mixed Greens
2ND NIGHT	Meat Loaf Florentine with Salsa	Rice with Grated Carrots
3RD NIGHT	Chicken Soup	Whole-grain bread
4TH NIGHT	Egg Fried Rice	
5TH NIGHT	🍲 Jamaican Roti	Mixed greens
GRAB & GO LUNCH	Second-Time Sloppy Joes	

🍲 = Second Supper recipe

WORK SCHEDULE

1 Clean and prep Crudités first so you can prep your carrots and celery for the soup at the same time.

2 Complete Chicken Soup and freeze in single-serving sizes.

3 Start rice for Rice with Grated Carrots to serve tonight with Meat Loaf Florentine.

4 Prepare meat loaf, wrap in foil, and bake. Freeze.

5 Marinate Jamaican-ish Pork until you are ready to bake for tonight's supper.

Crudités

SERVES: 4
PREPARATION TIME: 20 minutes

Cleaning and chopping *vegetables at the start of your cooking session means less work as you are in the process. Plus, it is always handy to have veggies ready when hunger hits.*

1 head celery
2 pounds carrots
1 each red and yellow bell peppers
1 head broccoli

◆ Clean the veggies and set aside 2 celery stalks and 4 carrots for soup as well as rice dish. Slice red and yellow bell peppers, broccoli, and remaining celery and carrots, and refrigerate in zip-top plastic bags with a piece of paper towel for up to 5 days.

TIPS

STORE VEGGIES IN a large freezer bag with one square of paper towel. Replace paper towel each time you open the bag as it absorbs the excess moisture, keeping veggies fresh longer.

Store peppers separately as they soften quicker and can hasten the spoilage of other vegetables.

Chicken Soup

SERVES: 4 as entrée +2 Grab & Go Lunches
PREPARATION TIME: 30 minutes

There's nothing more *comforting than chicken soup, especially when you feel a cold coming on.*

6 cups chicken stock (preferably homemade or frozen) (see Tip)
2 carrots
2 stalks celery
1½ pound boneless skinless chicken breast halves or thighs
1 onion, chopped
1 teaspoon garlic powder
1 teaspoon poultry seasoning
1 clove garlic, pressed
1 cup frozen corn niblets
1 cup frozen peas
Salt and pepper to taste

◆ In large saucepan, bring chicken stock to boil. Meanwhile, chop carrots and celery into small dice; set aside.

◆ Rinse chicken and cut into 1-inch pieces. Add to stock and simmer for 5 minutes. Skim foam from top.

◆ Add carrots, celery, onion, and garlic powder; simmer for 10 minutes.

◆ Add poultry seasoning and garlic. Stir in corn and peas; simmer 1 more minute. Add salt and pepper. (Refrigerate in small containers up to 3 days or freeze up to 1 month.)

THIS SOUP TRAVELS well either frozen so you can warm it up at work, or heated and carried in a Thermos. Take along an orange and a low-fat yogurt with the two remaining portions, and you have lunch.

TIP

FROZEN REAL CHICKEN stock is always best, but if you use the canned type be sure to add extra water to cut the salt.

Rice with Grated Carrots

SERVES: 4 as side dish + 4 for use in Second Supper
PREPARATION TIME: 5 minutes

This is the simplest rice recipe and it's as pretty as can be. Make it and store it in the fridge to serve with Meat Loaf Florentine and later fold into delicious Egg Fried Rice (see page 50).

3 cups chicken stock or water
1 ½ cups uncooked long-grain brown rice (see Tips)
2 carrots, grated
2 teaspoons fresh thyme leaves
½ teaspoon butter
Salt and pepper to taste

◆ In large saucepan, bring stock to boil. Add rice; cover and simmer for 30 to 40 minutes, or until tender and no liquid remains. Stir in carrots, thyme leaves, butter, salt, and pepper. Store 3 cups in a separate container to be used as a Second Supper in Egg Fried Rice.

To store, transfer to casserole dish; top with more grated carrot and sprig of thyme. Sprinkle with 1 teaspoon olive oil to keep top from drying out; place plastic wrap on top. Cover and refrigerate up to 24 hours.

TIPS

THIS RICE IS mild enough for fussy kids. To add a splash of spice, add 1 tablespoon Mexican Dressing (page 178).

Experiment with the brown rices now available, such as brown basmati, which cooks quickly. The short-grain brown sushi rice has a great stickiness that kids seem to like. Adjust cooking times according to package directions.

Egg Fried Rice

Leftover rice is perfect for Chinese stir-fried rice.

1 tablespoon canola oil, plus more as needed
1 clove garlic, minced
4 eggs
2 cups frozen peas
1 cup frozen corn niblets
1 carrot, grated
2 green onions, minced
3 cups cooked long-grain brown rice

HEAT 1 TABLESPOON canola oil in large skillet; add garlic and stir for 10 seconds, add eggs and scramble; remove to large bowl. Add peas to pan and cook until tender. Allow pan to reheat between additions and continue adding oil to cook one vegetable at a time. Fry rice last in small batches so it does not stick. (Unfortunately, this must be done with generous amount of oil and at high heat but adding lots of vegetables will balance the downside of this method.) Toss together ingredients in a bowl like a salad and sprinkle with soy sauce.

SERVES: 4 ➤ PREPARATION TIME: 10 to 12 minutes

Meat Loaf Florentine with Salsa

SERVES: 4 as entrée + 6 for Grab & Go Lunch
PREPARATION TIME: 20 minutes

Traditional meat loaf *has too much fat and no fiber. This version changes that with the additions of spinach and salsa.*

2 pounds lean ground beef
1 cup Italian-seasoned bread crumbs
¼ cup barbecue sauce or ketchup
2 eggs
3 tablespoons dried onion
2 tablespoons garlic powder
4 teaspoons dried oregano
2 tablespoons poultry seasoning
Salt and pepper to taste

TOPPING:
2 (10-ounce) packages frozen chopped spinach, thawed
1 cup grated Parmesan cheese
1 tablespoon dried oregano
Salt and pepper to taste
2 cups salsa

◆ In large bowl and using fork, mix beef, bread crumbs, barbecue sauce, eggs, onion, garlic powder, oregano, poultry seasoning, salt, and pepper. Divide and firmly pat into five foil mini loaf pans until each is two-thirds full.

◆ Topping: Squeeze as much liquid as possible from spinach; place in large bowl. Mix with Parmesan cheese, oregano, salt, and pepper. Divide and pat over meat mixture firmly with fork. Cover with foil.

◆ Preheat oven to 425°F. Place meat thermometer through foil and into center of one of the loaves without touching edges of pan. Bake loaves on baking sheet in 425°F oven for 1 to 1½ hours or until meat thermometer registers 170°F. Let cool for 20 minutes. Refrigerate for up to 3 days or freeze for up to 6 weeks.

◆ To reheat, thaw in fridge overnight. (Each loaf should serve two or three adults.) Bake in preheated 350°F oven for 45 to 60 minutes. Invert onto platter, cut into four slices. Serve with salsa on the side.

TIPS

IF YOUR KIDS don't like meat loaf, use an ice-cream scoop and serve in round balls called . . . meatballs. You could substitute ground pork, chicken, or turkey in this recipe; just scale up the bread crumbs a little to make sure the loaf is not too crumbly because the water content of these substitutes is higher.

Second-Time Sloppy Joes

DISGUISE THE BOUNTY of meat loaves you made. Thaw one loaf. Break up or chop into small pieces and stir into a pot containing about 3 cups of your favorite tomato sauce. Mash with a fork as it cooks and serve over whole wheat kaiser rolls.

COOKED, SLICED MEAT loaf is perfect in a sandwich. Round it out with a handful of the veggies that you prepared earlier in the week and an individual drink box of apple juice.

COOK ONCE A WEEK, EAT WELL EVERY DAY

Jamaican-ish Pork with Mixed Bean Salad and Greens

> **SERVES:** 4 as entrée + 6 for Second Supper
> **PREPARATION TIME:** 11 minutes

To make the *most of this dish in one go, bake all of the tenderloins and serve four people tonight, then chop the remaining pork and store it in the fridge to use as a Second Supper. Serve tonight's portion with mixed greens along with some whole-grain bread.*

2 teaspoons olive oil

6 cloves garlic, minced

3 tablespoons chopped fresh thyme (see Tip)

4 teaspoons chile powder

1 tablespoon allspice

1 tablespoon pepper

1 teaspoon ground cumin

¾ teaspoon salt

½ teaspoon ground cinnamon

½ teaspoon grated nutmeg

3 (12- to 16-ounce) pork tenderloins

1 (10-ounce package) prewashed mixed greens

1 (19-ounce) jar or can marinated mixed bean salad

1 loaf whole-grain bread, for serving

◆ In bowl, combine oil with garlic, thyme, chile powder, allspice, pepper, cumin, salt, cinnamon, and nutmeg; add pork, turning to coat. Transfer to three large zip-top plastic bags. Refrigerate one bag for up to 24 hours; freeze remaining two bags for up to 3 weeks. Thaw before cooking.

◆ Preheat oven to 450°F. Transfer pork from bag to roasting pan; roast in 450°F oven for 30 to 40 minutes until meat thermometer registers 160°F. Let stand for 5 minutes before cutting.

◆ Place the mixed greens in a large bowl and top with the mixed bean salad. Toss to combine. Serve with the pork and whole-grain bread.

TIP

FRESH THYME WILL keep for up to a month wrapped in plastic in the crisper of the fridge, but if you dry it, it will keep for up to 6 months in your cupboard. To dry, rinse thyme and pat dry with paper towel, then lay out on a baking sheet covered in foil. When you have finished baking the tenderloin, turn off the oven and place the thyme in the oven for up to 4 hours until dried. Then place the entire stems in zip-top plastic bags.

Jamaican Roti

1½ to 2 pounds reserved cooked pork
1 to 2 cups reserved mixed bean salad
4 Jamaican roti breads or other flatbread
2 cups frozen brussels sprouts
1 tablespoon bacon bits
1 teaspoon butter
Hot sauce, for serving

◆ Slice leftover pork into thin strips and toss with any remaining bean salad.
◆ In the meantime, steam or microwave brussels sprouts until soft, about 2 to 10 minutes.
◆ Toss the brussels sprouts with bacon bits and butter.
◆ Serve the pork mixture cold on a roti or other flatbread, with hot sauce. Serve brussels sprouts as a side dish.

SERVES: 4 ➤ **PREPARATION TIME:** 8 to 10 minutes

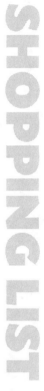

YOU NEED:

Baked Goods:

- ○ Whole-grain bread (1 loaf)
- ○ Italian-seasoned bread crumbs (1 cup)
- ○ 🥣 Whole wheat kaiser rolls (3)
- ○ 🥣 Whole-grain bread (18–24 ounce package)
- ○ 🥣 Roti or other flatbread (4 flatbreads)

Dairy:

- ○ Eggs (4)
- ○ Parmesan cheese, grated (1 cup)
- ○ Butter (1½ teaspoons)
- ○ 🥣 Low-fat yogurt (2 cups)

Meat and Alternatives:

- ○ Lean ground beef (2 pounds)
- ○ Pork tenderloins (three 12 to 16 ounce)
- ○ Boneless skinless chicken breasts or thighs (1½ pounds)

Produce:

- ○ Onion (1)
- ○ Mixed greens (10-ounce package)
- ○ Garlic (8 cloves)
- ○ Red bell pepper (1)
- ○ Yellow bell pepper (1)
- ○ Carrots (2¼ pounds)
- ○ Celery (2 heads)
- ○ Fresh thyme (¼ cup)
- ○ Oranges (2)
- ○ 🥣 Green onions (1 bunch)

Frozen Foods:

- ○ Frozen chopped spinach (two 10-ounce packages)
- ○ Frozen corn (2 cups)
- ○ Frozen peas (3 cups)
- ○ 🥣 Frozen brussels sprouts (2 cups)
- ○ Chicken stock (9 cups)

CHECK YOUR PANTRY FOR:

Condiments and Dressings:

- ○ Barbecue sauce or ketchup (¼ cup)
- ○ Salsa (2 cups)
- ○ Soy sauce (1 tablespoon)
- ○ 🥣 Hot sauce (1 small bottle)
- ○ 🥣 Bacon bits (1 tablespoon)

Cooking Oils:

- ○ Olive oil (1 tablespoon)
- ○ Canola oil (1 tablespoon)

Pastas and Tomato Products:

- ○ 🥣 Tomato sauce (two 18-ounce cans)

Canned Beans and Soup Broths:

- ○ Mixed bean salad (19-ounce jar or can)

Spices and Seasonings:

- ○ Poultry seasoning (7 teaspoons)
- ○ Dried onion (3 tablespoons)
- ○ Dried oregano (7 teaspoons)
- ○ Garlic powder (7 teaspoons)
- ○ Chile powder (4 teaspoons)
- ○ Allspice (1 tablespoon)
- ○ Ground cumin (1 teaspoon)
- ○ Ground cinnamon (½ teaspoon)
- ○ Grated nutmeg (½ teaspoon)

Grains:

- ○ Long-grain brown rice (1½ cups)

Juices:

- ○ Apple juice (2 single-serving juice boxes)

Dry Goods:

- ○ Mini foil loaf pans (5)

KEY: 🥣 denotes Second Supper or Grab & Go Lunch items

WEEK
4

SHOPPING LIST

Notes:

COOK ONCE A WEEK, EAT WELL EVERY DAY

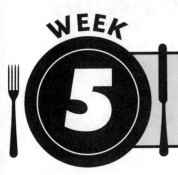

HAM BONE INTO HEARTY SOUP

WHEN I DISCOVERED that kale topped the list of healthy vegetables, I set out to make it palatable. I mean, let's face it, it's green, a little bitter, and smells strongly when cooked. One day I was drying herbs and a bunch of kale was just sitting there, on the verge of being released into compost heaven. What would I do with *it* if *it* were a batch of thyme that I pulled out of the garden just in time to build a snowman around it? I would dry it.

So I rinsed it, laid it out on a baking sheet, and sprinkled on some flavorings that are well liked in my house: chile powder, garlic, salt. I stuck it into the oven and walked the dog around the block. Upon my return, the house smelled slightly spicy and like roasted vegetables. To my surprise, the greens came up crispy and tasty. When I handed my daughter a bowl of this flaky green stuff as an afterschool snack (get 'em when they're hungry!), she daintily plucked out a leaf, then more heartily chomped on the rest of the bowl. You know the joy I am talking about, the relief, the high-fiving yourself in the kitchen when they actually eat something good for them.

We have since served this Krispy Kale as an hors d'oeuvre and have also crushed and sprinkled it on pasta for some color and flavor. When my daughter returns home to the smell of drying kale she actually cheers, "Yeah, kale!" I, of course, giggle inwardly while I admonish her not to eat too much and to leave some for the others.

WEEK 5 MENU CHART

SERVE	MAIN DISH	SERVE WITH
TONIGHT	Slow-Cooked Beer-Braised Beef	Red Pepper Rice, Lemony Steamed Broccoli
2ND NIGHT	Five-Spice Chicken with Hot Slaw	No extras necessary
3RD NIGHT	Chicken Fried Rice	No extras necessary
4TH NIGHT	Sunday Ham Soup with Romano Beans and Kale	Crusty whole-grain bread
5TH NIGHT	🥣 Vietnamese Five-Spice Soup	Mixed greens
GRAB & GO LUNCH	Beef Sandwich with Hot Mustard	
GRAB & GO LUNCH	Sunday Ham Soup with Krispy Kale	

🥣 = Second Supper recipe

WORK SCHEDULE

1 Simmer the ham bone for Sunday Ham Soup for up to three hours (as little as one hour will do in a pinch).

2 Brown the beef for the Slow-Cooked Beer-Braised Beef and continue with recipe until the pot goes into the oven.

3 Prepare broccoli to serve tonight with the beef but store in fridge covered in plastic until 10 minutes before supper. (Reserve two spears for lunch)

4 Make Red Pepper Rice.

5 Start Five-Spice Chicken with Hot Slaw to freezing point. Freeze for later in the week.

6 Complete Sunday Ham Soup.

Sunday Ham Soup with Romano Beans and Kale

> **SERVES:** 4 as entrée + 4 for Grab & Go Lunch
> **PREPARATION TIME:** 20 minutes

As with many *great discoveries, this was a happy accident. The smokiness of the ham high-lights the kale while the beans provide a soft comfort.*

    10 cups water
    1 ham bone, or pork hock
    2 cups any vegetable scraps (see Tips)
    1 dried ancho chile
    ½ cup orzo (see Tips)
    3 cups rinsed, coarsely chopped kale
    1 (19-ounce) can romano beans
    ¼ teaspoon ground cloves
    Crusty whole-grain bread, for serving

◆ In large pot, bring water, ham bone, vegetable scraps, and ancho chile to boil. Simmer for 1 to 3 hours (the longer, the more flavorful).

◆ Strain and return soup to pot, discarding ham bone, chile, and vegetables. (If spicy soup is desired, scrape out and discard seeds from chile; break chile into pieces and return to pot.) Freeze at this point (see Tip), or carry on with cooking instructions to serve within 4 days.

◆ Bring stock to boil; add orzo and cook for 5 minutes. Add kale, beans, and cloves; simmer for 5 minutes. Serve with crusty whole-grain bread. Freeze leftover soup in small containers (see Tips).

TIPS

THE HAM BONE AND vegetable scraps used in the recipe can come from Week 2 (see Tips, pages 26 and 29) or you could use any combination of onions/celery/carrots, but avoid broccoli and cauliflower as they are too sulfurous and take over the flavor. Or use whatever wilted vegetables you have on hand or have frozen over the week. Alternatively, you can purchase a prepack of "soup vegetables" at the supermarket.

Orzo is a rice-shaped pasta that is great as a side dish. Simply cook like other pasta and toss with butter, salt, pepper, and some grated Parmesan cheese.

Extras can be refrigerated up to 4 days but omit the orzo if you are going to freeze this dish, since pasta tends to get grainy and mushy as it continues to absorb liquid.

Sunday Ham Soup with Krispy Kale

◆ Reheat the soup and place each serving in a Thermos. Pack some cheese, crackers, and fruit for lunch, as well as some Krispy Kale.

◆ To prepare the Krispy Kale, rinse kale well under running water and pat dry with paper towels. Tear leaves into potato chip–size pieces; discard stems. Lay kale in single layer on one or two baking sheets. Sprinkle with chile powder, garlic powder, and salt to taste. Bake in a preheated 350°F oven until crisp but not browned, about 15 minutes. Turn oven off; leave kale in oven with door ajar until crisp and cool. Store in airtight containers. Serve as a side dish or appetizer.

SERVES: 6 ➤ PREPARATION TIME: 5 minutes

Slow-Cooked Beer-Braised Beef

SERVES: 4 as entrée + 2 for Grab & Go Lunch
PREPARATION TIME: 10 minutes

*T*his beef is *wonderful served with Lemony Steamed Broccoli and Red Pepper Rice (recipes follow). This can be prepared on the stovetop if you don't have a slow cooker.*

> 1 tablespoon canola oil
> 3 pound beef chuck roast
> 1 (12 oz.) bottle beer
> 1 onion, sliced
> 1 teaspoon soy sauce
> 1 teaspoon pepper
> 4 teaspoons dried basil

- ◆ If you don't have a slow cooker: Heat large pot over high heat; add oil. Brown roast on all sides. Add beer, onion, soy sauce, pepper, and basil; bring to boil. Cover and place pot in 275°F oven for 7 to 9 hours, or until meat is tender.
- ◆ To use a slow cooker: Omit oil and place beef directly into cooker. Top with remaining ingredients. Cook on high for 1 hour; reduce heat to low and cook for up to 8 hours.
- ◆ Store in fridge, sliced, with juices, for up to 3 days.

TIP

YOU CAN SERVE this with rye bread to sop up the juices. Be sure that rye flour is the first ingredient on the label, otherwise it is glorified white bread. Rye is lower on the glycemic index so it is absorbed more slowly by your body, which causes a slower rise in insulin.

Beef Sandwich with Hot Mustard

MAKE A SANDWICH with rye bread, hot mustard, leaf lettuce, and slices of the braised beef. Pack with 2 spears of broccoli and an orange juice box, to round out the meal.

SERVES: 1 to 3 ➤ **PREPARATION TIME:** 2 minutes

Lemony Steamed Broccoli

SERVES: 4
PREPARATION TIME: 5 minutes

When a steamer *is beyond your energy level, the microwave does a good job, fast.*

1 bunch broccoli, cut into florets (see Tips)
1 tablespoon white wine
1 teaspoon lemon juice
Pinch each salt and pepper

◆ Place broccoli in large microwavable bowl; sprinkle with wine, lemon juice, salt, and pepper. (Can be covered with plastic wrap and refrigerated up to 24 hours.)
◆ Microwave, covered, on high for 5 to 7 minutes until bright green and crisp-tender. Alternatively, you can steam the broccoli, covered, on the stovetop for 3 to 4 minutes.

TIPS

MANY GROCERY STORES carry packaged broccoli florets that are a time saver.

Even kids who don't like green vegetables may try them raw. Remember that kids need to see the same food anywhere from seven to twenty times before they will try it. Don't give up. Just keep putting out ridiculously small portions. Try serving broccoli in an eggcup filled with a spoonful of melted butter. Sometimes presentation goes a long way. A baby tree in the eggcup is worth two in the vegetable bin.

Red Pepper Rice

SERVES: 4 as entrée + 4 for Second Supper
PREPARATION TIME: 3 minutes

This is a *simple, microwavable side dish that you will use often.*

3 cups water
1½ cups uncooked brown basmati rice (see Tip)
1 teaspoon salt
1 red bell pepper
1 teaspoon unsalted butter
Pepper to taste

◆ In large microwavable bowl, combine water, rice, and salt; cover with plastic wrap. Core, seed, and grate red bell pepper into small bowl; cover with plastic wrap. Microwave rice on high for 15 minutes; fluff with fork and microwave on defrost level for 10 minutes or until tender. (Can be cooked on the stovetop. Bring rice and water to the boil, cover, reduce heat to medium, and simmer for 25 to 35 minutes.)

◆ Add red pepper, butter, and pepper; stir with fork, cover with plastic wrap, and let sit 5 minutes before serving. (Can be refrigerated for 24 hours.) Divide in half—serve half with Slow-Cooked Beer-Braised Beef and store the remainder for Chicken Fried Rice Second Supper.

TIP

BROWN RICE NEEDS to be a staple in your home; if you are having trouble making the switch, brown basmati is a good choice. It has more flavor and a less chewy texture than regular brown rice.

Chicken Fried Rice

1 tablespoon canola oil , plus more as needed
1 pound ground chicken
2 cups chopped celery
½ cup chopped broccoli
3 green onions, minced
2 to 3 cups reserved Red Pepper Rice
Soy sauce to taste
1½ cups cooked, cold brown basmati rice

◆ Heat 1 tablespoon canola oil in large skillet.
◆ Break ground chicken into skillet and stir-fry until fully cooked. Pour into a large bowl with all its liquid.
◆ Add chopped celery to skillet; stir-fry until tender and add to bowl. Stir-fry other veggies, reheating pan between additions and adding oil as needed.
◆ Fry rice last in small batches so it does not stick. Toss together ingredients in a bowl and sprinkle with soy sauce.

SERVES: 4 ➤ **PREPARATION TIME:** 15 to 18 minutes

Five-Spice Chicken with Hot Slaw

SERVES: 4 as entrée + 4 for Second Supper
PREPARATION TIME: 15 minutes

*G*rated cabbage isn't *just for coleslaw anymore. It is a healthy vegetable that goes well with Asian flavors—especially in this dish.*

18 skinless chicken drumsticks
½ cup low-sodium soy sauce
¼ cup brown sugar
2 tablespoons five-spice powder (see Tip)
1 (16-ounce) package coleslaw cabbage mix

◆ Rinse chicken and pat dry with paper towel; divide between two zip-top plastic bags.
◆ Add half each of the soy sauce, brown sugar, and five-spice powder to each bag; seal bags and rub on all sides to blend. Refrigerate to marinate at least 1 hour or up to 48 hours. (Freeze up to 3 weeks; thaw before proceeding.)
◆ Preheat oven to 400°F. Spread coleslaw mix on large foil-lined baking sheet; top with chicken and marinade. Bake in 400°F oven, uncovered, for 30 to 35 minutes, turning once, until juices run clear when chicken is pierced. Stir slaw if it starts to burn on edges.
◆ Once cooked, chicken legs can be frozen. Simply reheat in microwave for 3 to 5 minutes or serve cold with mixed greens. They're great for picnics.

TIPS

FIVE-SPICE POWDER is a great Chinese staple that usually can be found in supermarkets. If you can't find it, make your own with equal parts ground aniseed, ground ginger, ground cinnamon, and ground allspice. You can use five-spice powder in pumpkin pie or spice cookies; we used it once to spice up a chocolate cake and it was fabulous!

Vietnamese Five-Spice Soup

4 cups canned chicken broth

4 cups water

2-inch knob fresh ginger, halved

4 to 6 cooked, frozen Five-Spice Chicken legs, thawed

2 to 3 cups rice vermicelli or spaghettini

1 cup frozen green peas

2 to 4 tablespoon chopped fresh basil or mint leaves

◆ Stovetop method: Empty chicken broth and water into pot, add ginger and chicken legs, place lid on pot, and cook over high heat for 1 hour. Remove chicken and let cool just so you can slide meat from the bones, break into smaller pieces, and add back to the broth. Discard ginger. Add pasta and simmer on high until soft, about 3 minutes for rice or 6 minutes for spaghettini. Stir in peas and serve, topped with fresh basil or mint.

◆ Slow-cooker method: Empty chicken broth and water into pot, add ginger and chicken legs, cover, and cook on high for 1 hour. Reduce heat to low and let simmer 8 to 10 hours. Remove chicken and let cool just so you can slide meat from the bones, break into smaller pieces, and add back to the broth. Discard ginger. Add pasta and simmer on high until soft, about 30 minutes. Stir in peas and serve, topped with fresh basil or mint.

SERVES: 4 ➤ **PREPARATION TIME:** 25 minutes

YOU NEED:

Baked goods:
- ◯ 🍲 Rye bread (1 loaf)
- ◯ Crusty whole wheat bread (1 loaf)

Dairy:
- ◯ Butter (1 teaspoon)

Meat and Alternatives:
- ◯ Beef chuck roast (2 pounds)
- ◯ Skinless chicken drumsticks (18)
- ◯ 🍲 Ground chicken (1 pound)
- ◯ Ham bones—reserved from Week 1, or pork hock (1)

Produce:
- ◯ Red bell pepper (1)
- ◯ Kale (1 bunch)
- ◯ Celery (1 head)
- ◯ Coleslaw cabbage mix (16-ounce package)
- ◯ Mixed greens (10-ounce package)
- ◯ Dried ancho chile (1)
- ◯ Lemon juice (1 teaspoon)
- ◯ Onion (1)
- ◯ Broccoli (2 bunches)
- ◯ Green onions (3)
- ◯ 🍲 Fresh basil or mint (1 bunch)
- ◯ Leaf lettuce (3 leaves)
- ◯ 🍲 Gingerroot (2-inch knob)

Frozen Foods:
- ◯ 🍲 Green peas (1 cup)

CHECK YOUR PANTRY FOR:

Condiments and Dressings:
- ◯ Low-sodium soy sauce ($\frac{1}{2}$ cup plus 1 teaspoon)
- ◯ 🍲 Hot mustard (2 teaspoons)

Cooking Oils:
- ◯ Canola oil (2 tablespoons)

Pastas and Tomato Products:
- ◯ Orzo ($\frac{1}{2}$ cup)
- ◯ 🍲 Rice vermiccelli or spaghettini (3 cups)

Canned Beans and Soup Broths:
- ◯ Romano beans (19-ounce can)
- ◯ Chicken broth (4 cups)

Baking Products:
- ◯ Brown sugar ($\frac{1}{4}$ cup)

Spices and Seasonings:
- ◯ Five-spice powder (2 tablespoons)
- ◯ Dried basil (4 teaspoons)
- ◯ Ground cloves ($\frac{1}{4}$ teaspoon)
- ◯ 🍲 Chile powder (1 tablespoon)
- ◯ 🍲 Garlic powder (1 tablespoon)

Grains:
- ◯ Brown basmati rice ($1\frac{1}{2}$ cups)

Snack Foods:
- ◯ Rye crackers (1 package)

Juices:
- ◯ 🍲 Orange juice (4 single-serving boxes)

Beer and Wine:
- ◯ Beer 1 (12 ounce) bottle
- ◯ White wine (1 tablespoon)

KEY: 🍲 denotes Second Supper or Grab & Go Lunch items

SHOPPING LIST

Notes:

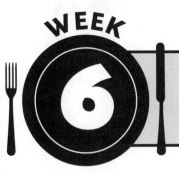

ADVENTUROUS OLDER KIDS

No ONE EVER cooks for me! When people find out what I do for a living they are hesitant to have me over to dinner. Listen up here and now, I will eat anything! Ask chefs what their favorite food is and they will all say eggs. We are so busy cooking and thinking about the next greatest thing that we crave the ease and versatility of something simple.

That said, it is always a good idea to have a few easy crowd-pleasers in your roster, one that's as good for company as it is for the kids. As the kids in the household get older, the difference between company food and family food gets smaller. The earlier you begin to experiment, the sooner this gap will close!

The Salmon with Spinach and Feta in Parchment is dead easy but looks as impressive as all get-out. I once suggested this meal for our "mumnet" (a mother's group I belong to) weekend away. Twenty mothers in a cottage gets pretty loud in the evening and lazy during the day. Sleeping in was strictly respected, so a no-fail, no-fuss recipe was a must. We prepared these packets assembly-line style and baked half in the oven and half on foil on the barbecue. We devoured the contents and threw away the wrappers so no one had to do the dishes. Perfect and peaceful.

WEEK 6 MENU CHART

SERVE	MAIN DISH	SERVE WITH
TONIGHT	Salmon with Spinach and Feta in Parchment	Polenta roll (optional)
2ND NIGHT	Chicken Breasts with Spicy Rub	Sesame Broccoli Salad and whole-grain bread
3RD NIGHT	Athenian Lamb and Lima Beans	Baked Mashed Potatoes and Potato Skins
4TH NIGHT	🍲 Fireside Supper	Cheese, crackers, pâté
5TH NIGHT	🍲 Apple Baked Schnitzel	Frozen green beans
GRAB & GO LUNCH	Celery Peanut Butter Logs	
GRAB & GO LUNCH	Honey Mustard Salmon Sandwich	

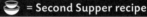 🍲 = Second Supper recipe

WORK SCHEDULE

1 Scrub and bake potatoes. Complete Baked Mashed Potatoes and Potato Skins to freezing point. Store in fridge or freezer.

2 Start lamb recipe up to first simmer, then turn off until later.

3 Complete Chicken Breasts with Spicy Rub and store in fridge until you are ready to cook tonight's supper.

4 Start Sesame Broccoli Salad and leave in fridge in covered bowl until ready to bake for tonight's supper.

5 Prepare salmon.

6 Finish Athenian Lamb and store in fridge or freezer for future use.

7 Clean celery for Celery Peanut Butter Logs, cut into sticks, and store in fridge, wrapped in paper towel, in zip-top storage bag.

Baked Mashed Potatoes and Potato Skins

> **SERVES:** 4 as side dish + 4 as part of Second Supper
> **PREPARATION TIME:** 15 minutes

Here's a side *dish and the foundation of a fun supper all in one.*

  6 medium-size baking potatoes (see Tip)
  ½ cup cream cheese
  2 teaspoons butter or margarine
  1 tablespoon dried rosemary
  1 teaspoon garlic powder
  Salt to taste

◆ Preheat oven to 450°F. Scrub potatoes; prick with fork in several places to let steam out so potatoes do not burst. Bake in 450°F oven for 45 to 60 minutes, or until tender.

◆ Let cool and cut in half; scoop insides into large bowl. Reserve skins with just enough potato in them to keep their shape, about ¼ inch.

◆ Add cream cheese and butter to the potatoes; mash with potato masher. Empty into greased casserole dish; cover with plastic wrap. Refrigerate for up to 3 days and serve with Athenian Lamb Stew, or freeze for up to 3 weeks. To reheat, thaw in refrigerator if frozen. Bake in preheated 450°F oven, uncovered, for 30 to 45 minutes until warmed through.

◆ Prepare the Potato Skins for Second Supper: Arrange potato skins on baking sheet, and sprinkle with rosemary, garlic powder, and salt. Cover and refrigerate for up to 3 days or freeze on sheet until solid, place in large zip-top plastic bags, and store in freezer for up to 3 weeks.

TIP

POTATOES HAVE RECEIVED a bad rap in recent years because they are a starchy food. However, the skin contains more potassium than a 6-ounce glass of orange juice and provides 19 percent of your vitamin B_6, as well as 10 percent of your magnesium for the day.

Fireside Supper or Porch Picnic

Kids love to simply change location once in a while, so use these potato skins as the foundation for a more casual meal. It may not feel like a meal to you but that is the whole point. Everyone will get fed, eat what they like, plus have a nutritious meal.

12 reserved Potato Skins
3 cups shredded Cheddar cheese
3 green onions, minced
2 cups salsa
4 stalks celery, sliced into sticks
2 cups baby carrots
1 (8-ounce) package whole-grain crackers
6 to 8 ounces chicken or pork liver pâté and vegetable pâté (see Tips)
4 ounces smoked salmon (optional)

◆ Preheat oven to 450°F. Place frozen skins in a single layer on a cookie sheet. Fill each skin with ⅛ to ¼ cup of shredded Cheddar cheese,
◆ Bake on baking sheet in oven for 10 to 20 minutes to melt cheese and crisp skins. Top with green onions and serve with salsa.
◆ As the skins reheat, put out a platter of celery sticks, carrots, and whole-grain crackers. Add a couple of pâtés (some of the veggie ones are great low-fat choices) or try smoked salmon.

SERVES: 4 ➤ PREPARATION TIME: 3 to 5 minutes

TIP

NOT ALL PÂTÉS are created equal. Read the ingredients before you buy, and try to find one that has chicken liver and/or pork liver as the first ingredient. After that, some have pork and egg whites as their bulk but others contain fat. Clearly pork and egg whites are the better, leaner, higher-protein choice. Veggie pâté is a great alternative made with soy, veggies, and seasonings—just be sure there is no hydrogenated vegetable oil or margarine in the ingredients.

Athenian Lamb and Lima Beans

SERVES: 4
PREPARATION TIME: 18 minutes

*L*amb **is a** *great alternative to beef. Ounce for ounce, it is comparable to the nutrition and fat content of beef, but since it is still naturally grass fed and not yet in the "machine raising" process that beef is, I tend to choose it over beef more often.*

2 teaspoons olive oil
12 ounces lean boneless lamb, cubed
1 onion, chopped
4 cloves garlic, minced
1 tablespoon dried oregano
Pinch hot pepper flakes
1 (19-ounce) can chopped tomatoes
½ teaspoon pepper
2 cups frozen lima beans, thawed
1 each red and yellow bell pepper, seeded, cored, and chopped
8 kalamata olives, rinsed
2 tablespoons capers, rinsed
¼ cup chopped fresh parsley
1 lemon, sliced

◆ In large ovenproof pot with lid, heat half the oil over high heat; brown lamb in batches. Transfer to plate.
◆ Add remaining oil to pan; reduce heat to medium. Add onion, garlic, oregano, and hot pepper flakes; cook, stirring, for 5 minutes or until softened.
◆ Return meat to pan along with any juices. Add tomatoes and pepper; bring to boil. Reduce heat, cover, and simmer for 30 minutes.
◆ Add beans, red and yellow bell peppers, olives, capers, and about ½ cup water to almost cover. Simmer over very low heat for 20 minutes, or until lamb is tender. (To store, cool in refrigerator and store for up to 3 days, or freeze for 1 month. Thaw in refrigerator overnight. Warm over medium heat.) Stir in parsley. Garnish with lemon slices.

Chicken Breasts with Spicy Rub

SERVES: 4 as entrée + 4 for Second Supper
PREPARATION TIME: 16 minutes

The "spicy" here refers to flavor, not heat, and you can increase or decrease the cayenne to alter the dish to your liking. Although the list of ingredients is long, don't be put off by it—this mix is a snap and will make a big batch of rub that can be stored in the fridge up to 1 month. It's a great last-minute rub for anything on the barbecue or in the oven. Try it on extra-firm tofu and pork or turkey cutlets.

Serve the chicken breasts with Sesame Broccoli Salad (page 76).

8 bone-in chicken breasts with skin (3 pounds, see Tip)

SPICY RUB:
¼ cup ground cumin
¼ cup packed brown sugar
2 tablespoons paprika
2 tablespoons black pepper
2 tablespoons red wine vinegar
2 tablespoons Dijon mustard
2 tablespoons canola oil
2 teaspoons cayenne pepper
2 teaspoons curry powder
2 teaspoons salt
1 teaspoon five-spice powder
4 cloves garlic, minced
2 to 4 tablespoons coconut milk (optional)

◆ Rinse chicken pieces under very cold water. Pat chicken dry with paper towel; set aside.
◆ Spicy Rub: In bowl, combine cumin, sugar, paprika, black pepper, vinegar, mustard, oil, cayenne pepper, curry powder, salt, five-spice powder, and garlic. Add desired amount of coconut milk, more for saucier dish. You could substitute water for a lower fat version. Smear all over chicken. (Refrigerate four breasts in zip-top plastic bag for up to 3 days and freeze remaining four for future use; thaw completely before baking.)
◆ Transfer to baking dish, and preheat oven to 325°F. Cover and bake in 325°F oven for 35 to 45 minutes, or until no longer pink inside. Uncover and bake 5 to 10 minutes to brown.

Apple Baked Schnitzel

*H*aving a rub in the fridge that is so versatile is a boon for the last-minute cook. Using the same rub here as in the recipe for Chicken Breasts with Spicy Rub, we net very different results. The first recipe uses a dry baking method and coconut milk but this second recipe uses a braising method with apple cider. The root vegetable chips are a welcome surprise and a healthy enough side dish if you keep the portions small.

4 tablespoons reserved spicy rub
4 pieces (about 1½ pounds) pork or turkey cutlets, or 8 ounces extra-firm tofu
1 cup apple cider or juice
3 cups frozen green beans
1 teaspoon butter
Salt and pepper to taste
1 (6-ounce) package root vegetable chips

◆ Preheat oven to 400°F. Rub Spicy Rub on both sides of cutlets. If using extra-firm tofu, slice in half horizontally to create a thinner piece and rub Spicy Rub on both sides.
◆ Place in large, low casserole dish, then pour apple cider over top.
◆ Bake in 400°F oven for 25 to 30 minutes.
◆ Steam green beans in microwave on high for 5 minutes or in a pot on the stovetop. Toss with butter and season with salt and pepper.
◆ Serve with root vegetable chips.

SERVES: 4 ➤ PREPARATION TIME: 6 minutes

Sesame Broccoli Salad

SERVES: 4 as side dish + 4 for Grab *&* Go Lunch
PREPARATION TIME: 20 minutes

Here's a unique *way to cook broccoli any time you have the oven on.*

> 2 heads broccoli
> ¼ cup sesame seeds, toasted (see Tips)
> ¼ cup rice wine vinegar
> ¼ cup low-sodium soy sauce
> 1 tablespoon olive oil
> 1 tablespoon toasted sesame oil
> 1 teaspoon grated gingerroot (see Tips)

◆ Preheat oven to 325°F. Wash broccoli. Break off florets; peel stems if desired and cut into 2-inch pieces. Place in bowl.

◆ In small bowl, combine sesame seeds, vinegar, soy sauce, olive oil, sesame oil, and gingerroot; pour over broccoli. Transfer broccoli to large baking sheet. Bake in 325°F oven for 30 minutes, or until broccoli is soft and soaks up some of the sauce. Serve warm or at room temperature.

TIPS

A JAR OF grated gingerroot lasts weeks in the fridge and does not develop an off-flavor like processed garlic. Use extras in a stir-fry. Or buy just 1 inch of the fresh root at the grocery store.

It's not necessary to toast sesame seeds but doing so provides a nuttier, headier flavor. Simply empty sesame seeds into a large skillet without oil and place over low heat for 5 to 10 minutes until they turn lightly brown, stirring often.

Salmon with Spinach and Feta in Parchment

SERVES: 4 as entrée + 2 for Grab & Go Lunch
PREPARATION TIME: 20 minutes

This dish has a great "wow" factor for when you have company. Substitute aluminum foil for the parchment if you prefer, but the parchment does make a nicer presentation.

2 (10-ounce) packages frozen chopped spinach, thawed
8 ounces light feta cheese, crumbled
1 clove garlic, minced
1 teaspoon dried oregano
4 (4- to 6-ounce) pieces fresh salmon fillet (plus 2 pieces as optional extras for lunch)
1 lemon, sliced
12 chives
Salt and pepper to taste

◆ Preheat oven to 400°F. Cut four pieces of parchment paper about 18 inches long. (Cut one extra piece if you are making leftovers for lunch.) Set aside.

◆ Squeeze as much water as possible from spinach; break up into bowl. Crumble feta into spinach; add garlic and oregano. Divide into four equal mounds; place each in center of parchment paper. Place piece of salmon on top of spinach. Top with slice of lemon and 3 chives. Sprinkle with salt and pepper. (For lunch portions, simply wrap together in parchment and bake as is; store in fridge until ready to make sandwiches.)

◆ Lift sides of parchment and fold accordion-style, leaving a couple of inches of space for heat to circulate; crimp edges and place on baking sheet. (Freeze in zip-top freezer bags for up to 2 weeks.) Bake on baking sheet in 400°F oven for 20 to 30 minutes from frozen, or 15 to 18 minutes if fresh, or until paper turns brown and puffy and fish flakes easily when tested with fork.

TIPS

FOR CHILDREN WHO are not keen on fish, add 1 tablespoon packed brown sugar and 1 teaspoon butter to each piece of fish. Omit spinach and add whatever vegetable they like: try grated carrots, sliced red bell pepper, or frozen green peas.

This meal stands alone without a starch side dish but, if you like, try a polenta roll. These rolls are made with whole-grain cornmeal and are normally sold in the deli section or near the dried pasta. They look like a big yellow sausage wrapped in plastic. Simply cut some slices, brush with olive oil, and bake on a baking sheet, uncovered, along with the salmon. The round yellow disks will complement the rectangular orange salmon.

If someone in your family hates salmon but you would like to serve this to the rest, simply substitute boneless skinless chicken breasts and proceed with the recipe. Increase baking time to 30 to 40 minutes.

Honey Mustard Salmon Sandwich

MASH REMAINING COOKED salmon with 2 tablespoons honey mustard and 2 tablespoons capers, and divide between 2 whole wheat hamburger buns. Wrap sandwiches tightly in plastic. Fill a plastic container with Sesame Broccoli Salad (page 76), and add a pear for a balanced lunch.

SERVES: 1 to 2 ➤ **PREPARATION TIME:** 2 minutes

Celery Peanut Butter Logs

Make sure these ingredients are on the table any time you think your kids will turn up their noses, and they will know they have an option to make themselves an alternative.

½ head celery, cut into stalks
½ cup peanut butter (see Tip)

◆ Clean celery stalks and let kids scoop their own peanut butter to fill the hollow. Serve with rye crackers and an apple.

SERVES: 4 ➤ **PREPARATION TIME:** 5 minutes

TIP

TRY SWITCHING TO almond butter once in a while. It has half of the fat, is never hydrogenated, and has twice the calcium of peanut butter.

YOU NEED:

Baked goods:
- ○ Whole-grain bread (1 loaf)
- ○ 🥣 Whole wheat hamburger buns (2)

Dairy:
- ○ Cream cheese ($^1/_2$ cup)
- ○ Light feta cheese (8 ounces)
- ○ Butter (3 teaspoons)
- ○ 🥣 Cheddar cheese, shredded (3 cups)

Meat and Alternatives:
- ○ Salmon fillet (four 4- to 6-ounce pieces, plus optional two extra pieces)
- ○ Smoked salmon (4 ounces) (optional)
- ○ Boneless lamb, cubed (12 ounces)
- ○ Chicken breasts, bone in (8 breasts, totaling 3 pounds)
- ○ 🥣 Pâté (two types, 4 to 6 ounces each)
- ○ 🥣 Pork cutlets or turkey cutlets (4 cutlets, totaling 1$^1/_2$ pounds)

Produce:
- ○ Green onions (3)
- ○ Red bell pepper (1)
- ○ Yellow bell pepper (1)
- ○ Onion (1)
- ○ Garlic (9 cloves)
- ○ Parsley (1 bunch)
- ○ Chives (1 bunch)
- ○ Gingerroot (1 teaspoon)
- ○ Celery (1 head)
- ○ Baking potatoes (6 medium-size)
- ○ Broccoli (2 heads)
- ○ Lemons (2)
- ○ 🥣 Pear (1)

- ○ 🥣 Apples (4)
- ○ 🥣 Extra-firm tofu (12 ounces) (optional)
- ○ 🥣 Baby carrots (2 cups)

Frozen Foods:
- ○ Frozen chopped spinach (two 10-ounce packages)
- ○ Frozen lima beans (2 cups)
- ○ 🥣 Frozen green beans (3 cups)

CHECK YOUR PANTRY FOR:

Condiments and Dressings:
- ○ Rice wine vinegar ($^1/_4$ cup)
- ○ Red wine vinegar (2 tablespoons)
- ○ Kalamata olives (8)
- ○ Capers (4 tablespoons)
- ○ Dijon mustard (2 tablespoons)
- ○ Honey mustard (2 tablespoons)
- ○ Salsa (2 cups)
- ○ Low-sodium soy sauce ($^1/_4$ cup)
- ○ Coconut milk (2 tablespoons) (optional)
- ○ Peanut butter (1 cup)

Cooking Oils:
- ○ Toasted sesame oil (1 tablespoon)
- ○ Canola oil (2 tablespoons)
- ○ Olive oil (4 teaspoons)

Pastas and Tomato Products:
- ○ Canned chopped tomatoes (19-ounce can)

Baking Products:
- ○ Brown sugar ($^1/_4$ cup)

Spices and Seasonings:
- ○ Sesame seeds ($^1/_4$ cup)

KEY: 🥣 denotes Second Supper or Grab & Go Lunch items

○ Curry powder (2 teaspoons)
○ Cayenne (2 teaspoons)
○ Five-spice powder (1 teaspoon)
○ Garlic powder (1 teaspoon)
○ Ground cumin ($\frac{1}{4}$ cup)
○ Hot pepper flakes ($\frac{1}{2}$ teaspoon)
○ Paprika (2 tablespoons)
○ Dried oregano (4 teaspoons)
○ Dried rosemary (1 tablespoon)

Snack Foods:
○ 🥣 Root vegetable chips, preferably made
with sweet potatoes (One 6-ounce
package)
○ 🥣 Whole-grain rye crackers (One 8-ounce
package)

Grains:
○ 🥣 Polenta roll (12 to 16 ounces) (optional)

Juices:
○ 🥣 Apple cider or juice (1 cup)

Dry Goods:
○ Parchment paper (1 package)

KEY: 🥣 denotes Second Supper or
Grab & Go Lunch items

Notes:

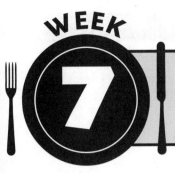

WEEK 7

HOUSEGUESTS!

SOMETIMES WE ARE called upon to juggle houseguests, their fussy kids, our fussy kids (with different fussiness, of course!), and our own desire to please and impress the adult palate. I take this challenge as an opportunity to include and expand everyone's tastes but I always have on hand a package or two of veggie dogs.

Part of my work involves teaching kids to cook (and taste). It's incredibly rewarding. They come with few preconceptions of how food should taste. I've found that once kids have invested effort in making a dish, they will be very interested in at least trying it when it's served. We encourage kids to try everything during class.

This week was designed with the help of my Kids Kan Cook class and has lots of options for leaving out spicy stuff when necessary. The squishy texture of the raw sausage in the Quick Italian Sausage and Kidney Bean Soup for this week put off a number of kids—until they smelled it cooking. The kidney beans were often left in the bowl but a few snuck into hungry mouths. The peppers became fun when one kid found a baby pepper inside her big one; pepper pearl diving became a sport that day.

The first time we make anything in class, it's all about exposure, not about how much gets eaten. Sausages become demystified, beans become not so bad, and peppers become downright fun. Only I know how much lycopene is in the tomato sauce, how much fibre is in the beans, and that the antioxidants in the peppers will be lifelong friends.

As usual, these recipes are mostly for four servings. Just scale up to accommodate houseguests.

WEEK 7 MENU CHART

SERVE	MAIN DISH	SERVE WITH
TONIGHT	Beef Tenderloin Steaks with Peppercorn Rub	Parmesan Barley Risotto and Baby Spinach Salad
2ND NIGHT	Quick Italian Sausage and Kidney Bean Soup	Whole-grain bread and cheese
3RD NIGHT	Crustless Broccoli and Cheese Quiche	Asparagus, toast
4TH NIGHT	🍲 Sausage and Sauerkraut on a Bun	Mixed greens
5TH NIGHT	🍲 Chinese Chicken with Green Beans and Broccoli	
GRAB & GO LUNCH	Italian Sausage and Kidney Bean Soup	
GRAB & GO LUNCH	Barley-Asparagus Salad	

🍲 = Second Supper recipe

WORK SCHEDULE

1 Rinse asparagus and set aside until ready to cook steaks.

2 Cook barley for Parmesan Barley Risotto and store in fridge for tonight.

3 Start Quick Italian Sausage and Kidney Bean Soup up to the simmer stage. Watch and turn off after 30 minutes until later.

4 Bake Crustless Broccoli and Cheese Quiches while soup and risotto simmer. Refrigerate or freeze.

5 Prepare Peppercorn Rub and rub beef tenderloin. Wrap well in plastic wrap; store in fridge until you are ready to cook tonight's supper.

6 Complete Quick Italian Sausage and Kidney Bean Soup.

COOK ONCE A WEEK, EAT WELL EVERY DAY

Asparagus in Its Own Juices

*A*lthough you'll want *to rinse the asparagus as the first step in this week's work schedule, you should finish the preparation just before you serve it—asparagus does not store well uncooked once the stems are cut and the lemon is added.*

1½ pounds fresh asparagus (the thinner the better)
1 tablespoon water
½ teaspoon salt
Pepper to taste
2 tablespoons unsalted butter (see Tip)
½ lemon

◆ Cut or break off tough bottom end of asparagus and discard. (Or freeze for soup scraps.) Rinse well under cold water, wrap in a clean tea towel, and store in fridge.
◆ Microwave instructions: Place asparagus on microwavable serving dish large enough to hold it slightly overlapping in sunburst pattern, tips facing in. Sprinkle with water, salt, and pepper; dot with butter. Squeeze lemon over top. Cover with vented plastic wrap. Microwave on high for 5 minutes until bright green. (Leftovers can be covered and refrigerated up to 3 days.)
◆ Stovetop steaming instructions: Bring 1 inch of water to a boil in a large low pot over high heat, add asparagus, cover, and steam for 3 minutes only. Lay on a platter in a sunburst pattern, squeeze lemon over, sprinkle with salt and pepper, dot with butter.

TIP

I SUGGEST USING unsalted butter in this dish, as it tends to be a fresher product (salt can mask stale flavors). Salt in butter also causes it to hold more water, which can affect your baking.

Parmesan Barley Risotto

> **SERVES:** 4 as side dish + 2 for Grab & Go Lunch
> **PREPARATION TIME:** 5 minutes

This risotto is *creamy and cheesy like the real thing, but replaces the traditional rice with a healthier grain. It is mild enough to sway the kids but interesting enough to please the adults.*

1 cup pot barley (see Tip)
3 cups chicken stock (preferably homemade or frozen)
¼ cup grated Parmesan cheese
Salt and pepper to taste

◆ In saucepan, simmer barley in chicken stock until tender, adding water if necessary, about 50 minutes. Drain any liquid. Transfer to microwavable dish; cool, cover, and refrigerate for up to 48 hours.

◆ To serve, microwave on high for 4 to 8 minutes until hot. Stir in Parmesan cheese, salt, and pepper. (Reserve 1 to 2 cups for Grab & Go Lunch; store in fridge, tightly covered.)

TIP

BARLEY IS HEALTHIER than rice or potatoes. Once your kids taste its chewy nuttiness, they will be more open to other more exotic grains. Try this recipe a couple of times before giving up. They may shun it at first but adding a little butter makes it taste like "baby popcorn."

Barley-Asparagus Salad

P**OUR** 2 TABLESPOONS olive oil and 1 tablespoon red wine vinegar over leftover barley, and chop and add any leftover asparagus. Toss in approximately ½ cup shredded Cheddar, salt, and pepper, and it becomes a great lunch salad. Serve with fruit juice box.

SERVES: 1 to 2 ➤ **PREPARATION TIME:** 3 minutes

Quick Italian Sausage and Kidney Bean Soup

SERVES: 4 as entrée + 4 for Second Supper (See Sausage and Sauerkraut on a Bun [page 86] for instructions on baking the balance of sausage)
PREPARATION TIME: 15 minutes

The chili-like flavors *in this soup make it a hit with most kids!*

Recipes like these, which can simmer for up to two hours, make the process of cooking many things at once possible. Try to find good beef stock in the freezer section of the grocery store. It is nutritionally superior to canned, and far less salty.

4 ounces Italian sausage (mild or spicy depending on the tolerance of the little ones) (see Tips)
1 large onion, finely chopped
2 cloves garlic, minced
2 green bell peppers, seeded and chopped
2 teaspoons Italian herb seasoning (see Tips)
2 (19-ounce) cans tomatoes, chopped
2 (19-ounce) cans tomato sauce
2 cups beef stock
1 cup dry red wine (optional)
2 (19-ounce) cans red kidney beans

◆ Remove casings and crumble sausage into a 3- to 4-quart saucepan. Cook over medium-high heat, stirring, until browned lightly. Add onion; cook until beginning to brown. Empty onto paper towel to drain off most of the drippings.

◆ Add garlic, green peppers, herb seasoning, tomatoes and their liquid, tomato sauce, beef stock, and wine. Return sausage mixture to pan and bring to boil; cover, reduce heat, and simmer 30 minutes. Stir in kidney beans and their liquid (which will thicken consistency of soup). If you like thinner soup, drain and rinse beans before adding.

Sausage and Sauerkraut on a Bun

This recipe will use up any leftover sausages you didn't cook for the Quick Italian Sausage and Kidney Bean Soup.

    1 pound Italian sausage
    1 (19-ounce) can sauerkraut
    1 tablespoon honey mustard
    1 (10-ounce) package prewashed mixed greens
    4 large submarine buns (whole wheat, if possible)

◆ While you have the package of sausage out, you may as well bake extras so they are ready for a quickie meal. Preheat oven to 400°F. Place all extra sausages on baking sheet lined with foil. Bake in 400°F oven for 15 to 25 minutes, depending upon the thickness of the sausages. Be sure they are firm and no longer pink. You may want to broil the sausages for 2 minutes at the end to give them that barbecued look.

◆ Drain and pat with paper towel before you store in a zip-top plastic bag in the fridge for 3 days or freezer for 3 weeks. They just need a quick zap in the microwave or 15 minutes in a preheated 400°F oven to reheat.

◆ Drain sauerkraut in a colander and run under cold water to remove some of the salt. The cabbage is a great, healthy vegetable, but the salt content detracts from its healthfulness. Place on each bun a sausage and some sauerkraut, some honey mustard, add a side salad and your car keys, and soccer night never looked so simple.

SERVES: 4 ➤ PREPARATION TIME: 8 minutes

Crustless Broccoli and Cheese Quiches

SERVES: 4 as entrée + 2 for Grab & Go Lunch (reheat as directed, and serve with some mixed greens and an orange)
PREPARATION TIME: 10 minutes

These mini quiches are great served with asparagus spears or a green salad. For kids who shun green, omit the broccoli and serve some fresh mint with the quiche instead. I've said it before: Mint has similar nutritional value to broccoli and even one leaf breaks down the myth that green stuff tastes bad. Let them pick a leaf or two and leave it at that for a couple of weeks. Step it up to fresh basil when they seem ready. In no time, they will try fresh baby spinach and then there is no stopping the great green giant!

2 teaspoons butter, or butter-flavored cooking spray
1 cup cream cheese
1 cup frozen broccoli
1 cup shredded Cheddar cheese
¼ cup milk
8 extra-large eggs
1 teaspoon dried oregano
¼ cup dry bread crumbs (optional)
4 sheets phyllo pastry (optional)

◆ Preheat oven to 425°F. Butter or spray six deep foil mini pie plates with cooking spray. Spread cream cheese evenly in bottoms of pans; set aside. Warm broccoli in microwave; press between paper towels until as dry as possible. Arrange over cream cheese.

◆ In large bowl, mix briskly with fork Cheddar cheese, milk, eggs, and oregano. Pour over broccoli.

◆ If desired, sprinkle pies with bread crumbs. Lay one corner of one phyllo sheet on top of each pie and spray with cooking spray or brush with butter. Fold in half and spray again. Fold into quarters and spray again. Scrunch up edges to fit dish. (Be sure to keep the open package of phyllo covered with a slightly damp cloth to prevent the dough from drying out.)

◆ Bake in 425°F oven for 30 minutes until just firm. (Let cool and freeze for 4 hours. Cover with foil and refrigerate up to 48 hours or freeze up to 3 weeks. To reheat, uncover and place in cold oven, then turn oven on to 350°F and bake for 30 to 40 minutes, just to warm through, or microwave on high for 2 minutes. The gentle warming prevents rubbery eggs.)

Beef Tenderloin Steaks with Peppercorn Rub

| SERVES: 4 |
| PREPARATION TIME: 10 minutes |

Serve with **Parmesan** *Barley Risotto (page 84) and baby spinach, which you can drizzle with Italian Dressing (page 178), if you'd like.*

3 teaspoons pepper
4 teaspoons ground ginger
2 teaspoons ground cardamom
4 cloves garlic, minced
½ cup low-sodium soy sauce
4 (4- to 6-ounce) boneless skinless chicken breasts, for Second Supper
4 (4- to 6-ounce) beef tenderloin grilling steaks (see Tips)
2 navel oranges
1 (8-ounce) package prewashed baby spinach (see Tips)

◆ In a large zip-top plastic bag, combine pepper, ginger, cardamom and garlic; mix in soy sauce. (Pour half into second bag and add boneless skinless chicken breasts, store in freezer until ready to use.) Add steaks to first bag and rub marinade all over steaks. (Leave children's portions plain if desired.) Store in fridge up to 24 hours. (Can be frozen for up to 3 weeks; thaw in refrigerator for 24 hours before cooking.)

◆ When ready to cook: Preheat oven to 425°F. Place thawed, marinated steaks on broiling pan. Slice oranges into wedges; store in covered bowl until ready for use.

◆ Roast steak on broiling pan, uncovered, in 425°F oven for 10 to 15 minutes, or until meat thermometer registers 140°F for rare or 160°F for medium.

◆ Arrange baby spinach on platter; top with steaks. Surround with orange wedges.

BAGS OF WHOLE-LEAF salad are better than cut-leaf salad, but they do go bad quickly once you open the bag. Don't be tempted to buy the lettuce from the open bins at the grocery store, since the factory packaging is more hygienic. (You never know whose hands have been in those bins.) To keep the bags fresher longer, roll leaves in a paper towel.

While a little more expensive, tenderloin steaks are uniformly tender and not at all gristly (the gristliness of some cuts of meat tends to turn kids off). Strip loin steaks are half the price and do almost as well here, but you will need to cut them down to size if you choose to substitute them.

You may omit the marinade for the kids but a little soy sauce will make for good color and flavor.

Chinese Chicken with Green Beans and Broccoli

4 marinated boneless skinless chicken breasts (reserved from Beef Tenderloin recipe, see page 88)
3 cups green beans, or yellow (wax) beans
2 heads broccoli
1 tablespoon canola oil
1 (8 ounce) package fresh Chinese vermicelli egg noodles

◆ Preheat oven to 375°F. Thaw frozen marinated chicken in microwave on a plate on defrost setting for 10 to14 minutes (or thaw in fridge overnight).

◆ Rinse green beans and broccoli under cold running water. Do not cut green beans but break off any tough stems or unsightly ends. Chop broccoli, very roughly, into 2-inch pieces. Toss broccoli and green beans in canola oil directly on cookie sheet or in large, low casserole dish. Top with chicken and its marinade, cover with foil, and bake at 375°F for 25 to 30 minutes until veggies are warmed through and chicken is cooked through and no longer pink.

◆ Meanwhile boil water and heat egg noodles according to package directions. Pile the noodles onto a serving platter and top with cooked chicken and vegetables.

SERVES: 4 ➤ **PREPARATION TIME:** 10 minutes

SHOPPING LIST

YOU NEED:

Baked goods:
- ○ Dry bread crumbs ($\frac{1}{2}$ cup)
- ○ Whole-grain bread (One 12- to 16-ounce loaf)
- ○ 🥣 Sandwich buns (4)
- ○ 🥣 Submarine rolls (4)

Dairy:
- ○ Eggs (8 extra-large)
- ○ Cream cheese (1 cup)
- ○ Milk ($\frac{1}{4}$ cup)
- ○ Unsalted butter (4 tablespoons)
- ○ Parmesan cheese, grated ($\frac{1}{4}$ cup)
- ○ 🥣 Cheddar cheese, shredded ($1\frac{1}{2}$ cups)

Meat and Alternatives:
- ○ Italian sausage ($1\frac{1}{4}$ pounds [🥣 including $\frac{1}{4}$ pound for Second Supper])
- ○ Beef tenderloin grilling steaks (four 4- to 6-ounce)
- ○ 🥣 Boneless skinless chicken breasts (four 4- to 6-ounce)

Produce:
- ○ Onion (1)
- ○ Mixed greens (10-ounce package)
- ○ Asparagus ($1\frac{1}{2}$ pounds)
- ○ Lemon ($\frac{1}{2}$)
- ○ Garlic (6 cloves)
- ○ Green bell peppers (2)
- ○ Navel oranges (4)
- ○ 🥣 Prewashed baby spinach (8-ounce package)
- ○ 🥣 Green beans or yellow (wax) beans (3 cups)

- ○ 🥣 Broccoli (2 heads [or 3 cups frozen])
- ○ 🥣 Chinese vermicelli egg noodles (8-ounce package)

Frozen Foods:
- ○ Phyllo pastry (4 sheets)
- ○ Frozen broccoli (1 cup, or 4 cups frozen if not using fresh)
- ○ Chicken stock (3 cups)

CHECK YOUR PANTRY FOR:

Condiments and Dressings:
- ○ Low-sodium soy sauce ($\frac{1}{2}$ cup)
- ○ 🥣 Red wine vinegar (1 tablespoon)
- ○ 🥣 Honey mustard (1 tablespoon)

Cooking Oils:
- ○ Canola oil (1 tablespoon)
- ○ Olive oil (2 tablespoons)

Pastas and Tomato Products:
- ○ Canned tomatoes (two 19-ounce cans)
- ○ Tomato sauce (two 19-ounce cans)

Canned Beans and Soup Broths:
- ○ Beef stock (2 cups)
- ○ Red kidney beans (two 19-ounce cans)
- ○ 🥣 Sauerkraut (19-ounce can)

Spices and Seasonings:
- ○ Dried oregano (1 teaspoon)
- ○ Ground ginger (4 teaspoons)
- ○ Italian herb seasoning (2 teaspoons)
- ○ Ground cardamom (2 teaspoons)

KEY: 🥣 denotes Second Supper or Grab & Go Lunch items

Grains:
- ⃝ Pot barley (1 cup)

Juices:
- ⃝ Orange juice (4 single-serving boxes)

Wine and Beer:
- ⃝ Dry red wine (1 cup) (optional)

Dry Goods:
- ⃝ Mini foil pie pans (6)
- ⃝ Large zip-top freezer bags (2)

Notes:

SHOPPING LIST

KEY: 🥣 denotes Second Supper or Grab & Go Lunch items

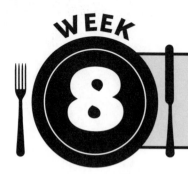

WEEK 8

CLASSIC COMFORT FOOD

I GREW UP with a French-Canadian mother who would often take my sisters and me back to her childhood home, the small town of Buckingham, Quebec. It was always a place of happiness, with cousins I could barely understand and lots of food. Ma Tante and Mon Oncle were like grandparents to me and Grandmère always smelled of home in the form of burnt toast. Here we used to sit down to a huge meal in the middle of the day, when the men would come home from the factory for lunch.

My entire morning was spent playing in the wide open field out back, with the smells of roasting meats and, my favorite, chicken stew and dumplings, wafting out through the window. We would sit down at a table stacked with every kind of comfort food you could imagine for twelve to eighteen people. The variety at each meal was endless and colorful. I learned to love potatoes in all their forms, and many vegetables free for the taking. There was never any comment about what we ate or did not eat, or how much of it was good for you. It was real, well-prepared food, and you would have to be crazy to turn your nose up at anything. It was also here that I learned to say yes to sugar pie and hide it in my room until I could make space for it in my full belly.

Gone are those easy, idyllic days in my fast-paced life, but I sure do close my eyes and imagine them every single time I eat Parsnip Puree Chicken Stew. It has all of the taste of Tante Louise's but none of the sins that you would expect from a French-Canadian kitchen.

WEEK 8 MENU CHART

SERVE	MAIN DISH	SERVE WITH
TONIGHT	Roast Beef with Rosemary and Garlic Veggies	No extras necessary
2ND NIGHT	Tuna Sailboats	Steamed Dilly Carrots
3RD NIGHT	Parsnip Puree Chicken Stew	No extras necessary
4TH NIGHT	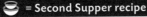 Beef and Pasta Toss	Romaine lettuce
5TH NIGHT	Pureed Carrot soup	Bagels with smoked salmon and low-fat cream cheese
GRAB & GO LUNCH	Tuna Roll-Ups	
GRAB & GO LUNCH	Parsnip Puree Chicken Stew	

= Second Supper recipe

WORK SCHEDULE

1. Cook Parsnip Puree Chicken Stew to simmer stage.

2. While chicken is simmering, prepare Tuna Sailboats and store in fridge or freezer.

3. Complete Parsnip Puree Chicken Stew and freeze.

4. Complete roast beef recipe up to and including refrigeration step until you are ready to cook tonight's dinner.

5. Steamed Dilly Carrots can be prepared and refrigerated until you are ready to cook Tuna Sailboats.

6. Clean romaine lettuce to serve with Beef and Pasta Toss and Tuna Sailboats, leave whole and store in fridge, wrapped in paper towel and stored in plastic.

Parsnip Puree Chicken Stew

SERVES: 4 as entrée + 2 for Grab & Go Lunch
PREPARATION TIME: 20 minutes

most stews are *thickened with flour but we use parsnips here for three reasons: to avoid the white flour starch, to add vitamins and fiber, and to add extra vegetables, which, since they are hidden, can't be picked out!*

> 2 pounds boneless skinless chicken thighs
> 2 teaspoons canola oil
> 1 medium-size onion, chopped
> 1 tablespoon butter
> 4 medium-size parsnips, peeled and cut into 2-inch pieces
> 2 stalks celery, chopped
> 1 teaspoon dried sage
> 1 teaspoon poultry seasoning
> 2 cups chicken stock (preferably homemade or frozen)
> 2 cups baby carrots, cut widthwise into thirds
> 2 cups frozen peas
> 4 small whole wheat or pumpernickel buns

- Rinse chicken and pat dry with paper towel; cut into 2-inch pieces.
- In large pot, heat oil. Stir in onion and cook on medium-high for 4 minutes. Add butter; brown chicken, in batches and without crowding the pan. Remove from pan and set aside.
- Add parsnip, celery, sage, and poultry seasoning to pot; stir for 30 seconds. Add stock and up to 2 cups water to just cover. Bring to boil; reduce heat to medium-low. Simmer for 12 to 15 minutes to soften parsnips. Using hand blender, puree into thicker, saucelike consistency.
- Add carrots and chicken; simmer 20 to 30 minutes until juices run clear when chicken is pierced. Add peas and warm through, 1 to 3 minutes. (Freeze up to 1 month. Thaw in refrigerator overnight. Microwave on high for 15 to 30 minutes, depending on serving size.)
- To serve, scoop out center of each bun; spoon stew into buns for a fun presentation.

FREEZE REMAINING PORTIONS of Parsnip Purée Chicken Stew in 1- to 2-cup containers, and reheat for lunch. Add a whole wheat bagel and a plum for a filling, nutritious meal.
SERVES: 1 to 2 ➤ **PREPARATION TIME:** 1 minute

Tuna Sailboats for Kids

SERVES: 4 as entrée + 4 for Grab & Go Lunch (see next recipe)
PREPARATION TIME: 10 minutes

While these **Tuna** *Sailboats are meant to be eaten with little hands, played with and enjoyed, adults can eat these like crabcakes on a bed of romaine lettuce with a squeeze of lemon.*

2 (7-ounce) cans tuna, drained
2 medium-size carrots, grated
2 eggs
2 cups dry whole wheat bread crumbs
¼ cup light mayonnaise (plus some for dipping if desired)
1 tablespoon olive oil
2 stalks celery
2 to 4 slices whole wheat tortillas
1 lemon

◆ In large bowl, mix tuna, carrots, eggs, bread crumbs, and mayonnaise until combined. Form into eight egg-shaped patties with dip in middle to make a fat "canoe." In nonstick skillet, heat oil; fry patties on both sides until golden. (Let cool; wrap separately and refrigerate for up to 2 days. Microwave on defrost for 2 to 5 minutes to warm through.)
◆ To serve, slice celery into thin sticks and tortillas into triangles. Cut slit into top of tortilla triangle. Let kids use the patty as a boat; at the table add a celery mast through the slit, and a tortilla sail.
◆ Adults can join the fun, or serve these to them as a "tuna cakes" salad, with a squeeze of lemon as dressing. A tiny dollop of extra mayo is always a treat.

Tuna Roll-Ups

FULL OF OMEGA-3 fatty acids, the tuna cakes are perfect for rolling into a whole wheat tortilla. Add some alfalfa sprouts and drizzle with a teaspoon of Italian Dressing (see page 178 for our recipe, or use store-bought) and serve with a pear for a satisfying, well-rounded meal.

SERVES: 1 to 2 ➤ **PREPARATION TIME:** 3 minutes

Roast Beef with Rosemary and Garlic Veggies

SERVES: 4 as entrée + 4 for Second Supper
PREPARATION TIME: 10 minutes

Every family seems to love roast beef night—together with roasted vegetables, it makes for a complete meal. Cutting the roast in half cuts down cooking time and ensures leftovers.

8 cloves garlic
2 tablespoons steak sauce
1 tablespoons Dijon mustard
1 sprig fresh rosemary, or 1 teaspoon dried
2 tablespoons olive oil
4 medium-size red new potatoes
1 cup baby carrots
1 medium-size red bell pepper, seeded, cored, and quartered
3 pounds sirloin tip oven roast, cut in half crosswise
½ cup beef stock (see Tips)
1 cup red wine (optional)

◆ Using garlic press, smash garlic. Add to large, shallow broiling pan. Mix in steak sauce, mustard, rosemary, and oil.

◆ Cut potatoes into quarters. Roll potatoes, carrots, and red peppers in oil mixture to coat. Spread out vegetables in pan, leaving space in center for the two pieces of meat.

- Smear meat with sauce mixture on bottom of pan. Pour in beef stock. (Cover and refrigerate up to 8 hours.)
- Place roasting pan in cold oven. Turn oven to 350°F; roast for 1 hour or until an instant-read thermometer reads 130°F to 135°F for medium-rare to medium.
- Transfer roast to cutting board; let stand for 5 minutes before carving. Slice up and place on a platter enough meat to serve four, then carve the leftovers into 1-inch strips to reserve for Beef and Pasta Toss (see below).
- Meanwhile, broil vegetables for 2 to 4 minutes until crispy, watching closely. Place vegetables on platter. Pour red wine into the roasting pan to deglaze it; stir and scrape up brown bits. Serve the pan juices with the roast beef and vegetables.

TIP

FREEZE REMAINING BEEF stock in ice cube trays. These are better than bouillon cubes and just as convenient to add to any sauce, soup, or even cooked rice. (An amazing treat for the family dog on a warm day!)

Beef and Pasta Toss

4 cups whole wheat penne
Reserved roast beef slices
1 (16-ounce) jar mild salsa
1 (8-ounce) jar marinated mushrooms
1 carrot, grated
¼ cup grated Parmesan cheese

- Cook whole wheat penne according to package directions; drain.
- Toss leftover meat with a mild salsa, marinated mushrooms, and a grated carrot.
- Toss pasta and meat together in a large bowl and top with Parmesan cheese just before serving.
- Complete the meal with a romaine lettuce salad on the side.

SERVES: 4 ➤ **PREPARATION TIME:** 8 minutes

Steamed Dilly Carrots

SERVES: 4 as side dish + 4 for Second Supper
PREPARATION TIME: 2 minutes

Two minutes prep *time gives you the fastest side dish around, and kids love these slightly sweet carrots.*

> 2 pounds baby carrots
> 3 tablespoons water
> 1 tablespoon liquid honey
> 1 teaspoon dried dill
> Pinch each salt and pepper

◆ Into large microwavable bowl, toss together carrots, water, honey, dill, salt, and pepper. Cover with plastic wrap. Microwave on high for 8 to 15 minutes, until crisp-tender. (Or place all the ingredients in a pot, add 1 inch of water, cover, and steam on the stovetop for 8 to 10 minutes.)

◆ Divide in half. Reserve second half for Pureed Carrot Soup for Second Supper. Store in fridge up to 3 days or in freezer up to 3 weeks.

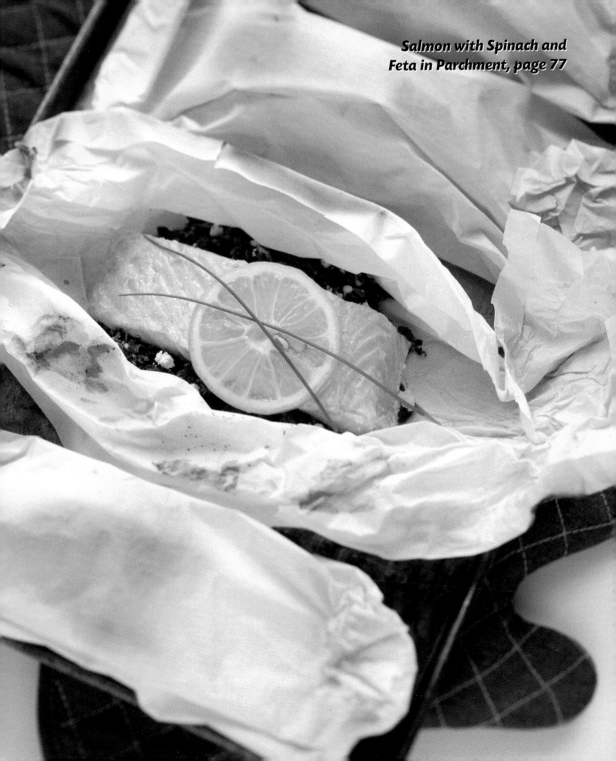

Salmon with Spinach and Feta in Parchment, page 77

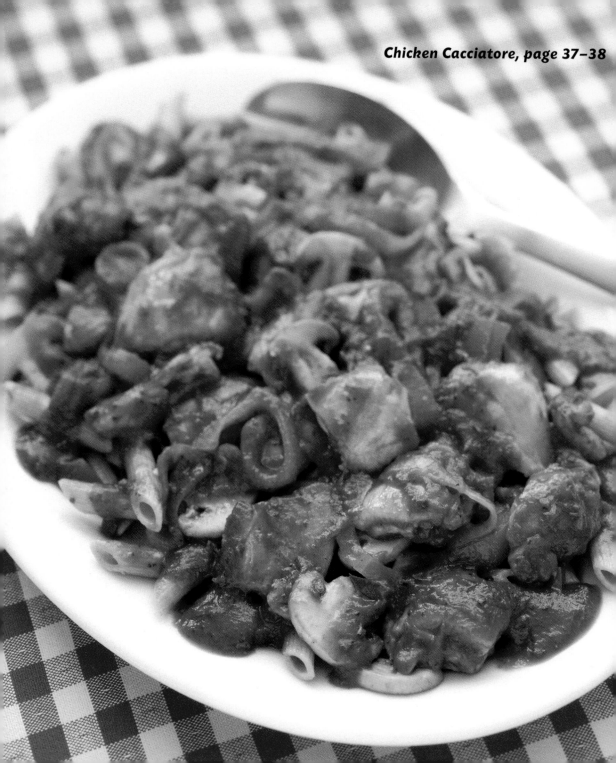

Chicken Cacciatore, page 37–38

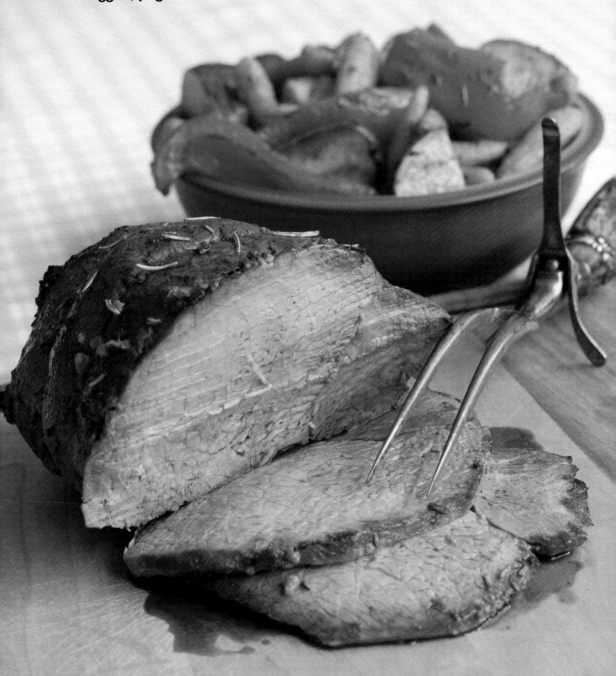

Roast Beef with Rosemary and Garlic Veggies, page 96

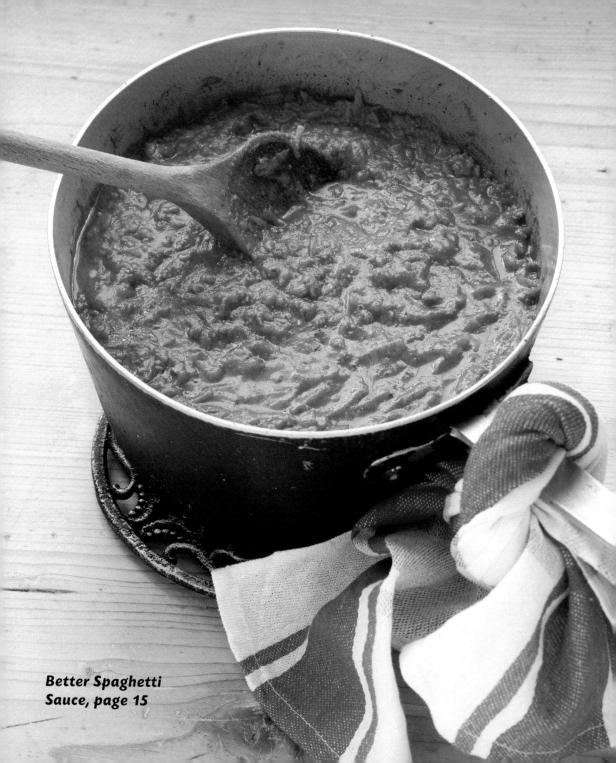

Better Spaghetti
Sauce, page 15

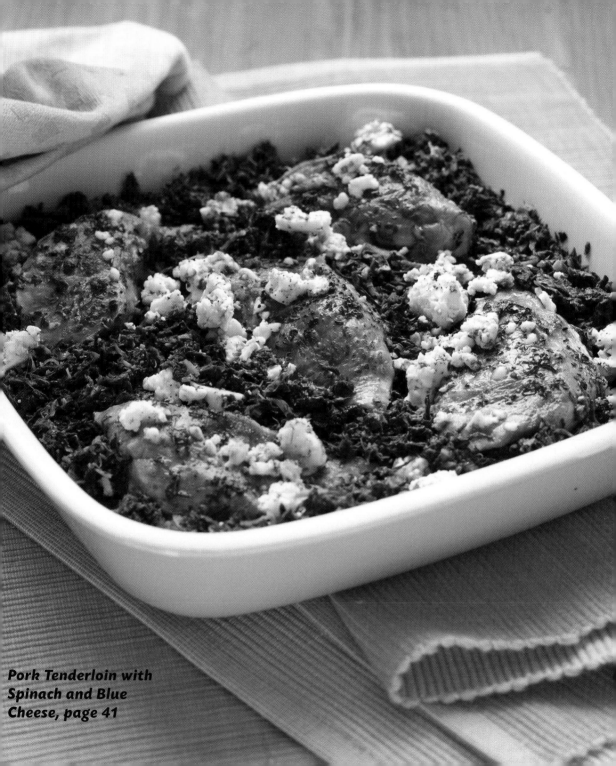

Pork Tenderloin with Spinach and Blue Cheese, page 41

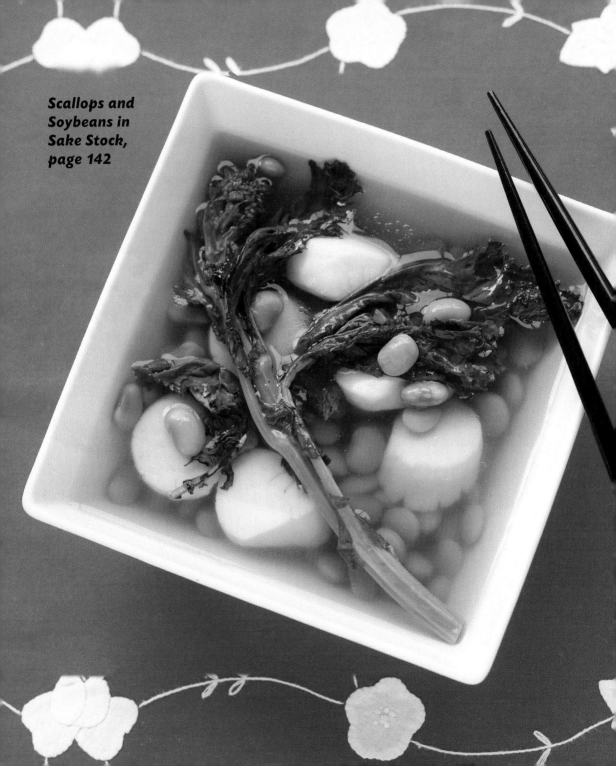

Scallops and Soybeans in Sake Stock, page 142

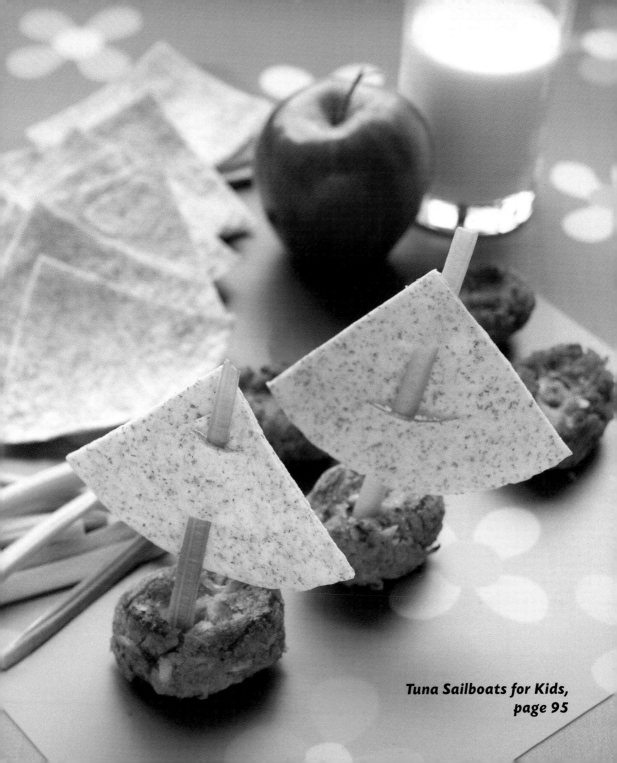

Tuna Sailboats for Kids,
page 95

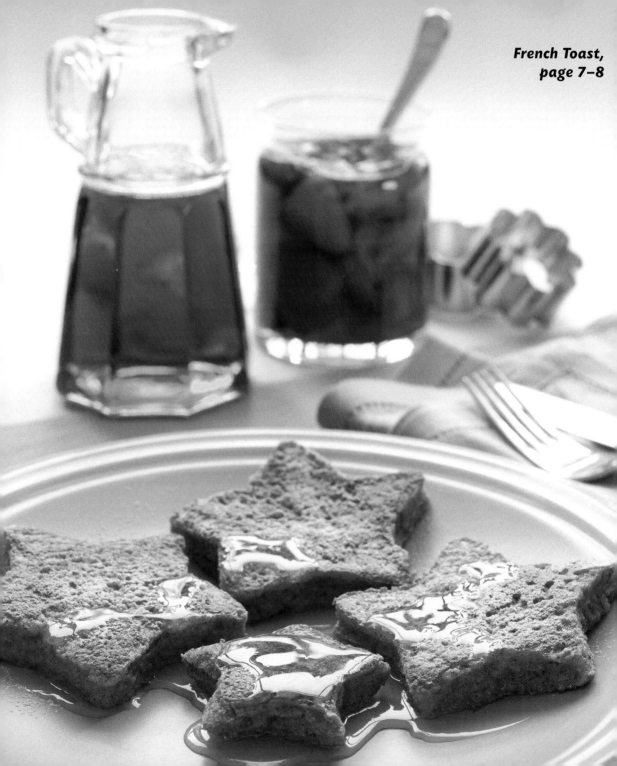

French Toast,
page 7–8

Pureed Carrot Soup

1 pound reserved, cooked Steamed Dilly Carrots
4 cups chicken broth (preferably frozen or homemade)
Honey, to taste
Salt and pepper, to taste
4 whole wheat bagels
4 ounces light cream cheese
6 ounces smoked salmon or 2 large ripe tomatoes (optional)
2 cups fresh snow peas, rinsed and dried
Mexican Dressing (see page 178)

◆ Place leftover cooked carrots in a large pot over medium-high heat. Add chicken stock and just enough water to cover.
◆ Bring to a boil, then puree the carrots with handheld blender and thin as desired with more stock and just enough honey, to make a slightly sweet thick soup. Depending on the stock, you may need to add salt and pepper.
◆ Serve with whole wheat bagels, cream cheese, and smoked salmon or ¼-inch thick slices of tomato. A side platter with raw snow peas with Mexican Dressing will set off these colors and flavors.

SERVES: 4 ➤ **PREPARATION TIME:** 15 minutes

YOU NEED:

Baked goods:
- ○ Whole wheat or pumpernickel buns (4)
- ○ Whole wheat tortillas (6)
- ○ Dry whole wheat bread crumbs (2 cups)
- ○ 🥟 Whole wheat bagels (6)

Dairy:
- ○ Eggs (2)
- ○ Butter (1 tablespoon)
- ○ 🥟 Parmesan cheese, grated (¼ cup)
- ○ 🥟 Cream cheese (4 ounces)

Meat and Alternatives:
- ○ Boneless skinless chicken thighs (2 pounds)
- ○ Sirloin tip oven roast (3 pounds)
- ○ 🥟 Smoked salmon (6 ounces, or substitute tomatoes [see below])
- ○ Tuna (two 7-ounce cans)

Produce:
- ○ Onion (1)
- ○ Parsnips (4)
- ○ Red new potatoes (4)
- ○ Carrots (3)
- ○ Baby carrots (3 pounds)
- ○ Celery (4 stalks)
- ○ Red bell pepper (1)
- ○ Garlic (8 cloves)
- ○ Fresh rosemary (1 sprig)
- ○ Lemon (1)
- ○ Romaine lettuce (1 head)
- ○ 🥟 Snow peas (2 cups)
- ○ 🥟 Plums (2)
- ○ 🥟 Pears (4)
- ○ 🥟 Alfalfa sprouts (1 pint)

- ○ 🥟 Beefsteak tomatoes (2) (optional)

Frozen Foods:
- ○ Frozen peas (1 pound)
- ○ Chicken stock (6 cups)

CHECK YOUR PANTRY FOR:

Condiments and Dressings:
- ○ Dijon mustard (1 tablespoon)
- ○ Steak sauce (2 tablespoons)
- ○ Light mayonnaise (¼ cup)
- ○ Honey (1 tablespoon, plus to taste)
- ○ 🥟 Marinated mushrooms (8-ounce jar)
- ○ 🥟 Mild salsa (16-ounce jar)

Cooking Oils:
- ○ Olive oil (3 tablespoons)
- ○ Canola oil (2 teaspoons)

Pastas and tomato products:
- ○ 🥟 Whole wheat penne (1 pound)

Canned Beans and Soup Broths:
- ○ Beef stock (½ cup)

Spices and Seasonings:
- ○ Poultry seasoning (1 teaspoon)
- ○ Dried sage (1 teaspoon)
- ○ Dried dill (1 teaspoon)

Wine and Beer:
- ○ Red wine (1 cup) (optional)

KEY: 🥟 denotes Second Supper or Grab & Go Lunch items

Notes:

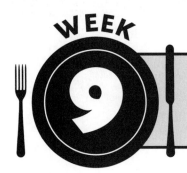

WEEK 9

ALMOST VEGETARIAN

ONCE, WHEN I had five vegetarian houseguests, I abandoned them all to go out to a party at my publishers. My guests dined on what I had left behind.

The people I met at the party that night were all impressed that I could calmly talk about the future of this book while I had a hungry houseful, but I have always been most comfortable being well ahead of schedule. As my husband has finally learned, 6:00 or 6:30 means 5:59 to me. Being prepared is more than just the Girl Scout's law, it is the mother's credo. When the foundations of a meal are made, then anyone can warm it up and put it on the table. Guilt disappears as the ice melts off the frozen Molasses Lentil Soup. Peace sets in when Tofu Caesar Salad needs only a bag to be opened and a toss to its leaves. Harmony happens when your guests ask for the recipe because their kids prompted them to do so. Business (studies, groceries, laundry, PTA . . .) is well under way when our lives are nourished with good food and great friends—who don't mind feeding themselves once in a while.

Scale up recipes to serve all your houseguests.

SERVE	MAIN DISH	SERVE WITH
TONIGHT	Lemony Baked Shrimp	Poppy Seed Noodles, Asian Sprout and Red Pepper Salad
2ND NIGHT	Molasses Lentil Soup	Curried Tortilla Crisps
3RD NIGHT	🥣 Grilled Chicken Caesar Salad	Whole-grain bread
4TH NIGHT	Easy Minestrone	Tofu Caesar Salad
5TH NIGHT	🥣 Lentil Quesadillas	Smoked Almond and Apple Salad
GRAB & GO LUNCH	Molasses Lentil Soup	
GRAB & GO LUNCH	Protein Poppy Seed Noodles	
GRAB & GO LUNCH	Tofu Sprout Salad	

🥣 = Second Supper recipe

WORK SCHEDULE

1 The Molasses Lentil Soup and Easy Minestrone can be cooked at the same time in two separate pots, which saves steps. Chop and cook two onions together and then divide into two large pots, then continue on with the Molasses Lentil Soup recipe.

2 When you get to the stage of simmering lentils, start on Easy Minestrone. Complete both soups and store in freezer in serving sizes that you will use. For instance if you sit together as a family, one large container will do, but if you eat at different times, perhaps single-serving sizes makes more sense.

3 Complete Poppy Seed Noodles and store in fridge, covered.

4 Mix Tofu Caesar Salad dressing and store in fridge up to one week. Prepare and store greens.

5 Assemble Lemony Baked Shrimp; cover and store in fridge up to 6 hours until you are ready to bake for tonight's supper.

6 Toss together Asian Sprout and Red Pepper Salad and refrigerate, covered, until suppertime.

Molasses Lentil Soup

SERVES: 4 as entrée + 4 for Second Supper + 2 for Grab & Go Lunch
PREPARATION TIME: 18 minutes

The sweetness of *this soup has converted many a lentil hater. Serve with tortillas sprayed with oil and sprinkled with curry powder and salt, then baked in 400°F oven for 20 minutes while you reheat soup.*

2 teaspoons canola oil
1 onion, chopped (see Tips)
2¼ cups dried red lentils (see Tips)
2 red potatoes, diced
2 carrots, diced
8 cups vegetable stock or water
1 cup frozen corn niblets
1 tablespoon dried oregano
2 cups tomato or V-8 juice
¼ cup lemon juice (optional)
3 tablespoons molasses (see Tips)
Salt and pepper to taste

◆ In very large pot, heat oil. Add onion; cook for about 4 minutes to soften.
◆ Stir red lentils, potatoes, and carrots into onions. Add vegetable stock and bring to boil. Reduce heat and simmer 15 minutes.
◆ Remove 1¼ cups of cooked lentils to a plastic container and store as is in the fridge for up to 4 days for Second Supper, Lentil Quesadillas.
◆ Add corn, oregano, tomato juice, lemon juice if desired, and molasses. Bring to simmer; cover and simmer 5 minutes. Add salt and pepper.
◆ Refrigerate up to 4 days or freeze up to 6 weeks. Store any leftover soup in 1 to 2-serving size containers, for Grab & Go Lunch.

REHEAT INDIVIDUAL PORTIONS of soup. Round out with snow peas and a container of fruity low-fat yogurt on the side.
SERVES: 1 to 2 ➤ **PREPARATION TIME:** 2 minutes

Lentil Quesadillas with Smoked Almond and Apple Salad

4 (10-inch) whole wheat tortillas
1¼ cups reserved cooked lentils
1 cup grated mozzarella cheese
4 teaspoons dried oregano (or to taste)
1 teaspoon garlic powder (or to taste)
1 teaspoon dried hot chile peppers (or to taste)
Cooking spray
6 cups prewashed mixed greens
1 ripe avocado
4 tablespoons salsa
4 ounces smoked almonds
 2 Red Delicious apples, sliced
4 dashes bottled lime juice

◆ Preheat a nonstick skillet while you lay out tortillas on a clean counter. Top half of each tortilla with one-quarter of the reserved lentil mixture, placing it off center so you can fold in half easily. Top each with approximately ¼ cup grated mozzarella, and sprinkle each with oregano, dried garlic, and chile peppers. Fold in half and place into hot nonstick skillet that has been sprayed with cooking spray. Cook over high heat for 2 to 3 minutes per side, two at a time. Remove to cutting board and let sit to cool before slicing into two large triangles. Continue with remaining quesadillas.

◆ Meanwhile, set out four plates with one-quarter of the mixed greens on each plate. Top each with ¼ avocado, sliced, 1 tablespoon salsa, 1 ounce smoked almonds, and ½ sliced apple. Squeeze a dash of lime juice over all.

SERVES: 4 ➤ PREPARATION TIME: 12 to 15 minutes

Easy Minestrone

SERVES: 4 as entrée + 4 for Grab & Go Lunch
PREPARATION TIME: 20 minutes

The amount of *ground beef called for in traditional minestrone recipes often adds a lot of unnecessary fat and calories; and the pasta in typical minestrone doesn't do well in the freezer. This recipe addresses both issues and so becomes a healthier, low-calorie choice that's great right out of the freezer.*

1 tablespoon olive oil
1 cooked, chopped onion (from Molasses Lentil Soup, page 104) or 1 onion, chopped
2 carrots, chopped
2 stalks celery, chopped
½ each red and green bell pepper, seeded, cored, and chopped
2 cloves garlic, minced
2½ to 3 cups vegetable stock or chicken stock
3 cups canned, chopped stewed tomatoes
1 leek (white and light green part only), washed well and chopped into rings
1 (19-ounce) can mixed beans, drained and rinsed
1 cup frozen peas
3 tablespoons store-bought pesto sauce (see Tip)
4 tablespoons plain low-fat yogurt (optional)

◆ In large stockpot, heat oil and cooked onion over medium heat (or, heat oil; add chopped onion and cook until softened, about 4 minutes). Add carrots, celery, and red and green bell peppers, stirring after each addition. Add garlic, stock, and tomatoes; bring to boil over high heat. Reduce heat, cover, and simmer for 20 minutes or just until vegetables are tender.

◆ Add leek and beans; simmer for 2 minutes. Stir in frozen peas and pesto. (Refrigerate up to 5 days or freeze up to 1 month. Be sure to store four portions of soup in single-serving size containers so you can enjoy for Grab & Go Lunch.) Serve with a dollop of low-fat yogurt, if desired.

Poppy Seed Noodles

SERVES: 4 as side dish + 4 for Grab & Go Lunch
PREPARATION TIME: 2 minutes

Using egg noodles *in this dish boosts the protein.*

4 cups dried egg noodles
2 tablespoons poppy seeds (see Tips)
1½ tablespoons toasted sesame oil
Salt and pepper to taste

◆ In large pot of boiling salted water, cook noodles until just tender; drain. Add poppy seeds and oil; toss to coat. Season with salt and pepper to taste.

◆ Refrigerate up to 2 days; serve cold or reheat in microwave for 2 minutes.

◆ Set aside half of the noodles for Grab & Go Lunch.

Protein Poppy Seed Noodles

½ recipe cooked Poppy Seed Noodles
2 cups silken tofu, mashed

T OSS THE RESERVED noodles with 2 cups mashed silken tofu to make a complete protein. Serve cold with a cubed mango or peach. Red bell pepper sticks are a nice addition.

SERVES: 4 ➤ **PREPARATION TIME:** 2 minutes

Tofu Caesar Salad

SERVES: 4 as side dish + 4 for Second Supper + 2 for Grab & Go Lunch
PREPARATION TIME: 3 minutes

Caesar salad is *a favorite for many kids. They tend to like its creamy texture and salty nature, but we could all do without the fat-laden mayonnaise that many bottled and home recipes use. We have tried this tofu version on many Caesar-loving adults and kids, and they can't taste the difference—but their bodies notice! Be sure to use the anchovy; it adds calcium and good oils. Fresh lemon juice and excellent olive oil will make it even better.*

½ cup silken tofu
2 tablespoons grated Parmesan cheese, plus extra for serving
2 tablespoons lemon juice
2 dashes Worcestershire sauce
1 clove garlic, minced
2 dashes Tabasco sauce
1 tablespoon extra-virgin olive oil
1 tablespoon white wine vinegar
1 teaspoon mashed anchovies or anchovy paste, optional (see Tip)
Salt and pepper to taste
2 heads romaine lettuce
3 slices cooked bacon (or simulated bacon bits made from soy)

◆ In bowl, mash together tofu, Parmesan cheese, lemon juice, Worcestershire sauce, garlic, Tabasco sauce, oil, vinegar, anchovies, salt, and pepper. Let sit for 1 hour. (Can be stored in fridge for up to 1 week. Dressing does not freeze well.)

◆ Clean and dry the lettuce. Leave one head intact as full leaves until you are ready to use for Grilled Chicken Caesar—roll it in paper towel and store in plastic bag until ready to use. Tear the remaining head of lettuce into pieces, and roll in paper towel and store in plastic bag until ready to use.

◆ Toss the torn lettuce with 4 tablespoons dressing; top with cooked bacon or simulated bacon bits and pass extra Parmesan cheese at the table.

Grilled Chicken Caesar Salad

Though there is tofu in the dressing as protein, adding a few ounces of chicken will make this salad into an even more substantial meal.

> 1 pound boneless skinless chicken breasts
> ¼ cup barbecue sauce
> Reserved Caesar Salad dressing
> Reserved, cleaned romaine lettuce from Tofu Caesar Salad

◆ If the chicken breasts have been frozen, place them on a microwave-safe dish and thaw in the microwave on defrost setting until soft throughout. Once thawed or if starting from refrigerated: switch to high setting and partially cook for about 12 to 15 minutes on high. (Pour juices down the drain and rinse clean sink and plate thoroughly with hot soapy water.)

◆ Preheat broiler. Pour barbecue sauce over the chicken and broil on high, about 4 inches from the heat for 4 minutes per side, until chicken is no longer pink inside.

◆ Slice the chicken into strips; arrange over romaine lettuce tossed with 4 tablespoons Tofu Caesar salad dressing.

SERVES: 4 ➤ **PREPARATION TIME:** 7 to 10 minutes

Lemony Baked Shrimp

> **SERVES:** 4
> **PREPARATION TIME:** 8 minutes

Serve with *Poppy Seed Noodles (page 107). This is a nonvegetarian option for this week. Vegetarians can eat the Protein Poppy Seed Noodles (see page 107).*

> 2 pounds frozen medium-size raw shrimp, peeled and deveined
> ³⁄₄ cup dry bread crumbs
> 2 tablespoons finely chopped fresh parsley
> 1 teaspoon grated lemon zest
> ¹⁄₂ teaspoon salt
> 6 cloves garlic, minced
> ¹⁄₄ cup lemon juice
> 4 teaspoons olive oil

◆ Preheat oven to 400°F. Coat four individual gratin dishes with cooking spray. Divide shrimp among dishes.
◆ In bowl, combine bread crumbs, parsley, lemon zest, salt, and garlic; stir in lemon juice and oil. Sprinkle evenly over shrimp. (Refrigerate up to 6 hours.)
◆ Bake in 400°F oven for 15 to 30 minutes (will take up to 30 minutes if shrimp cooked from frozen, or as little as 15 minutes if they were thawed in refrigerator), or until shrimp are pink and opaque.

TIPS

FRESH PARSLEY CAN be stored in a glass of water in the refrigerator up to 10 days. You can put it out on the table so anyone can pick a leaf and sprinkle it over dinner. When it starts to dry out, then help it dry all the way by spreading on a cookie sheet and baking in 200°F oven for an hour or so. Store dried parsley as you would any other spice in the cupboard up to 6 months.

The peel-and-eat aspect of shrimp doesn't appeal to everyone, so be sure to buy shrimp that has been peeled but frozen raw, if your family does not like peeling.

You can substitute 2 pounds halibut, cut into 2-inch cubes, for the shrimp. Do not mix with the remaining ingredients until just before baking because the tenderness of the fish can't take the acid of the lemon and will get mushy.

Asian Sprout and Red Pepper Salad

This is a colorful and simple addition to any meal. Serve with Lemony Baked Shrimp (page 110).

1/4 cup low-sodium soy sauce
1/4 cup toasted sesame oil
2 tablespoons grated gingerroot
2 tablespoons rice wine vinegar
4 cups bean sprouts
1 red bell pepper, thinly sliced or grated

◆ In small bowl, whisk together soy sauce, sesame oil, ginger, and vinegar; set aside.
◆ Rinse sprouts very well under cold running water. Drain well and place in bowl. Add dressing and red pepper; toss to coat well. (Can be refrigerated up to 3 days.)

Tofu Sprout Salad

CUBE 1 CUP of firm tofu and toss with extra sprout salad. Let sit to marinate at least 1 hour before serving. This is a nice light meal for a hot day with a cool, cubed mango and a mango-flavored yogurt drink.
SERVES: 1 to 3 ➤ **PREPARATION TIME:** 6 to 8 minutes

SHOPPING LIST

YOU NEED:

Baked goods:
- ◯ Dry bread crumbs (³/₄ cup)
- ◯ Whole-grain bread (1 loaf)
- ◯ Whole wheat tortillas (eight 10-inch)
- ◯ Whole wheat crackers (8 ounce package)

Dairy:
- ◯ Parmesan cheese, grated (2 tablespoons)
- ◯ Plain low-fat yogurt (4 ounces)
- ◯ Fruity low-fat yogurt (4 single-serving tubs)
- ◯ Mango-flavored yogurt drink
- ◯ Mozzarella cheese, grated (1 cup)

Meat and Alternatives:
- ◯ Cooked bacon (3 slices) (optional)
- ◯ Boneless skinless chicken breasts (1 pound)

Produce:
- ◯ Silken tofu (2¹/₂ cups)
- ◯ Lemon juice (³/₄ cup)
- ◯ Grated lemon rind (1 teaspoon)
- ◯ Red potatoes (2)
- ◯ Carrots (4)
- ◯ Green bell pepper (¹/₂)
- ◯ Red bell peppers (1¹/₂)
- ◯ Celery (2 stalks)
- ◯ Romaine lettuce (2 heads)
- ◯ Gingerroot (2 tablespoons)
- ◯ Garlic (9 cloves)
- ◯ Leek (1)
- ◯ Onions (3)
- ◯ Fresh parsley, finely chopped (2 tablespoons)

- ◯ Bean sprouts (4 cups)
- ◯ Snow peas (2 cups)
- ◯ Mango or peach (1)
- ◯ Firm tofu (1 cup)
- ◯ Mixed greens (6 cups)
- ◯ Avocado (1)
- ◯ Red Delicious apples (2)

Frozen Foods:
- ◯ Frozen shrimp, medium-size raw, peeled (2 pounds)
- ◯ Frozen peas (1 cup)
- ◯ Frozen corn niblets (1 cup)
- ◯ Vegetable stock (8 cups)

CHECK YOUR PANTRY FOR:

Condiments and Dressings:
- ◯ Mashed anchovies or anchovy paste (1 teaspoon)
- ◯ Pesto sauce (6 tablespoons)
- ◯ Worcestershire sauce (2 dashes)
- ◯ Tabasco sauce (2 dashes)
- ◯ Lime juice (4 dashes)
- ◯ White wine vinegar (1 tablespoon)
- ◯ Low-sodium soy sauce (¹/₄ cup)
- ◯ Rice wine vinegar (2 tablespoons)
- ◯ Barbecue sauce (¹/₄ cup)

Cooking Oils:
- ◯ Extra-virgin olive oil (1 tablespoon)
- ◯ Olive oil (4 teaspoons)
- ◯ Canola oil (2 teaspoons)
- ◯ Vegetable oil cooking spray
- ◯ Toasted sesame oil (¹/₃ cup)

KEY: denotes Second Supper or Grab & Go Lunch items

Pastas and Tomato Products:

○ Tomato or V-8 juice (2 cups)

○ Canned, chopped stewed tomatoes (3 cups)

○ Egg noodles (4 cups dried)c

○ 🥘 Salsa (4 tablespoons)

Canned Beans and Soup Broths:

○ Mixed beans (19-ounce can)

○ Vegetable stock (3 cups)

Baking Products:

○ Molasses (3 tablespoons)

Spices and Seasonings:

○ Dried oregano (2 to 3 tablespoons)

○ Poppy seeds (2 tablespoons)

○ Curry Powder (1 tablespoon)

○ 🥘 Garlic powder (1 teaspoon)

○ 🥘 Dried chile peppers (1 teaspoon)

Snack Foods:

○ 🥘 Smoked almonds (6 ounces)

Legumes:

○ Red lentils ($2\frac{1}{4}$ cups dried)

Notes:

KEY: 🥘 denotes Second Supper or Grab & Go Lunch items

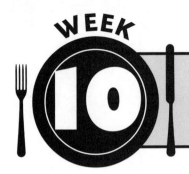

I MEET A lot of parents who worry that their kids eat like birds. "Just wait," I tell them. Kids don't need a lot of calories to get through the day when they are little, and, if they know how to say no when they are full (instead of listening to you urging them to clean their plates), they will be well prepared for the battle against adult indulgence.

Of course, there is some singing that goes on in the heart when you see a kid hunker down to a good meal. When they are truly hungry and there is no stopping them, be sure to have good food ready. They will blast through your kitchen like the Tasmanian Devil. We used to watch my nephew at about age twelve eat cereal from a salad bowl. He could down a box of shredded wheat in two days. We could not keep our place stocked with enough food when he was around. And then his friends would come over! Now at over six feet tall, he can still out-eat his dad, but he's a healthy, strapping example of good food in, good kid out.

In one cooking class, I had a preteen along with the others who were age seven to nine. The younger ones began to insist that we put his portion of our just-cooked food on a separate plate, because he could demolish the platter before any of them could even reach it.

Your kids will eat—eventually. Focusing on lifelong habits rather than the number of corn niblets ingested helps. And keeping the teenagers at the back of the line at any family function will be something you'll have to get used to soon enough.

WEEK 10 MENU CHART

SERVE	MAIN DISH	SERVE WITH
TONIGHT	Souvlaki Pork with Tossed Greek Salad and Yogurt Feta Dip	No extras needed
2ND NIGHT	Lower-Fat Chili con Carne	Mixed greens with Mexican Dressing
3RD NIGHT	Chicken Stuffed with Sun-Dried Tomatoes and Chèvre	Quinoa and Carrots
4TH NIGHT	🍲 Chili Pie	Corn, salsa
5TH NIGHT	🍲 Creamy Chicken Soup with Goat Cheese	Whole-grain bread, sun-dried tomatoes, avocado
GRAB & GO LUNCH	Chili Wraps	
GRAB & GO LUNCH	Pork Picnic	
Grab & Go Lunch	Quinoa Feta Salad	

🍲 = Second Supper recipe

WORK SCHEDULE

1. Sauté ground beef for Lower-Fat Chili con Carne while you wash and prepare veggies for the chili and the souvlaki.

2. Drain and complete chili recipe once you have removed all vegetables from the sink.

3. Assemble Chili Pie and Chili Wraps, wrap tightly in plastic and store in fridge up to 4 days.

4. Chop and marinate pork for souvlaki for 4 to 8 hours, and serve tonight.

5. Chop veggies for Tossed Greek Salad. Make dip.

6. Assemble Chicken Stuffed with Sun-Dried Tomatoes and Chèvre.

7. Clean and chop Crudités to get a head start on the week for lunches.

8. Quinoa and Carrots can be prepared on the day you cook the Chicken Stuffed with Sun-Dried Tomatoes and Chèvre.

Lower-Fat Chili con Carne

SERVES: 4 as entrée + 4 for Second Supper + 2 for Grab & Go Lunch
PREPARATION TIME: 20 minutes

By **running hot** *water over the cooked ground beef we take out a lot of extra fat. Adding lots of vegetables updates this family pleaser, which is perfect served with mixed greens and Mexican Dressing (see page 178).*

1 pound ground beef (such as chuck)
2 cups chopped onion
2 stalks celery, chopped
2 green bell peppers, seeded, cored, and chopped
2 tablespoon finely minced garlic
2 tablespoon chile powder
1 teaspoon dried oregano
1 teaspoon ground cumin
¼ teaspoon pepper
1 bay leaf
1 (6-ounce) can unsalted tomato paste (see Tips)
3 cups canned, chopped tomatoes
¾ cup water
1 tablespoon red wine vinegar
1 (19-ounce) can red kidney beans, drained
1 tablespoon Chile Spice (page 175) (optional)

◆ In large, deep pot, sauté beef until no longer pink. Pour into colander and drain off fat. Run hot water over meat; let sit in sink to remove even more fat.

◆ Add onion, celery, and green pepper to pot; cook until onion is translucent, 6 to 8 minutes. Add garlic, chile powder, oregano, cumin, pepper, and bay leaf; stir for 1 minute. Return meat to pan; add tomato paste, canned tomatoes, water, and vinegar. Bring to boil; reduce heat and simmer 15 minutes.

◆ Stir in beans; simmer 15 minutes. Remove bay leaf before serving.

◆ Stir in Chile Spice if desired. (Freeze in single-serving containers for up to 6 weeks.) Set aside half to use in Second Supper and Grab & Go Lunch. Or you could assemble the Chili Pie (page 117) as well as a few burrito wraps (page 118) and store in the fridge or freezer.

Chili Pie

Try to find soft corn tortillas for this, as they use the whole grain and have a dense texture that is crispy when baked. If you can't find them, whole wheat flour tortillas are a good substitute. Add a mixed green salad.

> 4 (10-inch) soft corn tortillas
> 2 to 3 cups reserved Lower-Fat Chili con Carne
> 1 (18-ounce) jar salsa
> ½ cup shredded Cheddar cheese
> 3 to 4 cups frozen corn niblets, for serving

◆ Preheat oven to 350°F. Oil a round casserole dish and lay a corn tortilla on the bottom.

◆ Warm chili in the microwave (or on the stovetop) and spread on the tortilla. Place a second tortilla on top and spread with ¼ cup salsa, repeat with the third and fourth tortilla. Sprinkle the fourth tortilla with shredded cheese. (You can prepare and refrigerate this for up to 2 days before serving, but it takes mere minutes to assemble if you want to make it just before dinner.)

◆ Bake 30 to 45 minutes, uncovered. Slice into triangles and serve like a pizza, with frozen corn that has been heated, and any extra salsa.

SERVES: 4 ➤ **PREPARATION TIME:** 5 minutes

Chili Wraps

IMMEDIATELY WRAP ANY remaining chili in whole wheat tortillas and roll up burrito style. Wrap up each burrito in plastic wrap and place in the refrigerator for up to 3 days, so individual lunches are ready to go. Pack some cucumber and some Yogurt Feta Dip (below) as a side dish, along with some fruit.

SERVES: Varies ➤ **PREPARATION TIME:** 5 minutes

Souvlaki Pork with Tossed Greek Salad and Yogurt Feta Dip

SERVES: 4 as entrée + 4 for Grab & Go Lunch
PREPARATION TIME: 15 minutes

Serve this with some mixed greens and whole wheat pita pockets. There is enough dip / dressing here to serve you throughout the week and, if you don't have to share with Super Bowl guests, you will have a bunch of lunches under your belt.

SOUVLAKI:

2 pound pork tenderloin

¼ cup olive oil

1 clove garlic

1 teaspoon dried oregano

Salt to taste

½ lemon

SALAD:

1 cucumber

1 red bell pepper

3 stalks celery

½ cup pitted black olives, preferably kalamata

YOGURT FETA DIP:

> 2 cups plain low-fat yogurt
> ¼ cup crumbled feta cheese
> 1 tablespoon honey Dijon mustard
> 1 teaspoon garlic powder
> 1 teaspoon dried oregano
> Salt to taste

◆ Souvlaki: Cut pork into 2-inch cubes; place in large zip-top freezer bag. Add oil, garlic, oregano, and salt. Squeeze the juice from the half lemon into bag and throw in the lemon rind. Seal bag and shake. Refrigerate to marinate up to 24 hours. (Meat can be frozen up to 3 weeks; thaw in refrigerator.)

◆ Salad: Cut cucumber, red bell pepper, and celery into cubes; toss with olives.

◆ Dressing/Dip: In bowl, mix yogurt, feta cheese, Dijon mustard, garlic powder, oregano, and salt. Drizzle a few tablespoons over the cucumber mixture and toss to coat; serve the rest as a dip.

◆ Preheat oven to 450°F. Arrange pork in single layer in roasting pan; bake in 450°F oven for 16 to 18 minutes, until just a hint of pink remains inside. Broil for 1 to 2 minutes to brown. Serve family style on a platter so everyone can serve themselves.

TIP

IF YOUR KIDS are very particular about foods touching each other then lay the salad out on a platter and cover with plastic wrap. Leave olives in a separate dish for adults to enjoy.

Pork Picnic

ONCE THE PORK is cooked, you can freeze it to serve as eat-on-the-run finger food with some carrot and celery sticks. Freeze it for up to 3 weeks and thaw in the fridge. Serve cold or warmed in microwave on defrost setting for a few minutes. Add one or two slices of whole wheat tortilla.

SERVES: Varies ➤ **PREPARATION TIME:** 2 to 3 minutes

Chicken Stuffed with Sun-Dried Tomatoes and Chèvre

SERVES: 4 as entrée + 4 for Second Supper
PREPARATION TIME: 8 minutes

Food, like fashion, *has its time. But some things last: the pairing of tomatoes and chèvre—goat cheese—has become a timeless classic. Delicious!*

> 10 sun-dried tomatoes packed in oil (see Tips)
> 1 tablespoon light mayonnaise (optional)
> 2 cloves garlic, minced
> 6 ounces chèvre
> 1 teaspoon crumbled dried rosemary
> Salt and pepper to taste
> 8 boneless skinless chicken breasts (3 pounds)

◆ Chop tomatoes roughly.
◆ In bowl, mix together mayonnaise if using, tomatoes, garlic, chèvre, rosemary, salt, and pepper.
◆ Pat chicken dry with paper towels. Lay out four large pieces of plastic wrap about 18 inches long; place 2 breasts on each. Scoop about 1 tablespoon cheese mixture onto each breast. Fold breasts around cheese mixture envelope-style and turn over. Smear remaining cheese mixture on each breast. Wrap plastic around each pair. Place packages in large zip-top freezer bag. (Store in freezer up to 3 weeks.)
◆ Preheat oven to 350°F. In plastic wrap, partially precook 4 breasts in microwave for 10 to 15 minutes on high. Remove plastic wrap and place in baking dish, leaving space between each.
◆ Bake in 350°F oven for 25 to 35 minutes, or until no longer pink inside. Serve with Quinoa and Carrots (page 122).

TIP

YOU CAN ALSO use dry-packed tomatoes, which will reduce the fat content of this dish. Place them in a microwavable dish, cover with water, and microwave on high for 5 minutes; drain and chop.

Creamy Chicken Soup with Goat Cheese

This soup is fantastic with a side salad of avocado and cherry tomatoes drizzled with balsamic vinegar and olive oil. If you want to get a head start on the preparation, place the broth, water, and potatoes in a slow cooker and set on low before you go out for the day. They will be ready to puree at suppertime and all you will need to do is chop the chicken and allow it to reheat in the soup.

> 4 cups chicken broth (preferably homemade or frozen)
> 2 cups water
> 3 unpeeled new potatoes, scrubbed and chopped into 2-inch pieces
> 1 teaspoon dried thyme
> 2 to 4 reserved Chicken Breasts with Sun-Dried Tomatoes and Chèvre, roughly chopped
> Skim milk to thin soup
> Salt and pepper to taste
> Extra chèvre and chopped sun-dried tomatoes (optional), for garnish

◆ In saucepan, bring chicken stock with water to boil.

◆ Add the potatoes and dried thyme; simmer over medium heat until potatoes are tender, about 15 minutes.

◆ Using hand blender, puree until smooth; add chicken and return to boil. Reduce heat and simmer until chicken is warmed through, 2 to 3 minutes. Add some milk to thin to desired consistency, but do not boil or it will separate. Add salt and pepper to taste, and top with more chèvre and sun-dried tomatoes if you like.

SERVES: 4 ➤ **PREPARATION TIME:** 10 minutes

Quinoa and Carrots

SERVES: 4 as side dish + 2 for Grab & Go Lunch
PREPARATION TIME: 4 minutes

This is a *great side dish to prepare the day you cook your Chicken Stuffed with Sun-Dried Tomatoes and Chèvre. Quinoa may be somewhat unfamiliar, but it has more magnesium, zinc, copper, and iron than brown rice and cooks in a third of the time. Once you try this teensy-weensy powerhouse with butter, you will get over its weird name, which is pronounced "keenwa."*

2 cups water or chicken stock
1 cup dried quinoa
2 cups frozen sliced carrots
1 tablespoon butter
Salt and pepper to taste

◆ In large pot, bring water to boil. Add quinoa; cook for 10 minutes until quinoa breaks up a bit.

◆ Meanwhile, microwave carrots just to thaw. Add to quinoa; simmer 2 to 5 minutes until softened and warmed through. Stir in butter, salt, and pepper. (Refrigerate up to 24 hours.)

Quinoa Feta Salad

CHOP SOME FRESH green beans into leftover quinoa and add 2 to 3 ounces of cubed feta cheese. Drizzle with 1 tablespoon or so of balsamic vinegar to make a hearty salad. Pack a cup of grapes and a juice box for a light but filling lunch.

SERVES: Varies ➤ **PREPARATION TIME:** 5 minutes

TIPS

IF YOU WANT TO skip the new grain or just can't find it at the grocery store, substitute such small pasta as orzo (cook it according to package directions before proceeding with the recipe).

YOU NEED:

Baked goods:
- ○ Whole wheat pita bread (8)
- ○ 🍚 Whole wheat tortillas (10)
- ○ 🍚 Corn tortillas (4)
- ○ 🍚 Whole-grain bread (1 loaf)

Dairy:
- ○ Soft chèvre (6 ounces)
- ○ Feta cheese ($1/2$ cup)
- ○ Plain low-fat yogurt (2 cups)
- ○ Butter (1 tablespoon)
- ○ 🍚 Cheddar cheese, shredded ($1/2$ cup)
- ○ 🍚 Skim milk ($1/4$ to $3/4$ cup)

Meat and Alternatives:
- ○ Pork tenderloin (2 pounds)
- ○ Ground beef chuck (1 pound)
- ○ Boneless skinless chicken breasts
  (8, totaling 3 pounds)

Produce:
- ○ Sun-dried tomatoes, oil packed or
  dehydrated (10)
- ○ Red bell pepper (1)
- ○ Green bell pepper (2)
- ○ Onions (2)
- ○ Garlic (5 cloves)
- ○ Cucumber (2)
- ○ Celery (7 stalks)
- ○ Mixed greens (two 10-ounce packages)
- ○ Lemon ($1/2$)
- ○ Baby carrots (1 pound)
- ○ 🍚 New potatoes (3)
- ○ 🍚 Avocado (2)
- ○ 🍚 Cherry tomatoes (2 pints)

- ○ 🍚 Green beans (1 cup)
- ○ 🍚 Red grapes (2 cups)
- ○ 🍚 Bananas (2)

Frozen Foods:
- ○ Frozen sliced carrots (2 cups)
- ○ 🍚 Frozen corn (3 to 4 cups)
- ○ 🍚 Chicken stock (6 cups)

CHECK YOUR PANTRY FOR:

Condiments and Dressings:
- ○ Honey Dijon mustard (1 tablespoon)
- ○ Light mayonnaise (1 tablespoon) (optional)
- ○ Black olives ($1/2$ cup)
- ○ Red wine vinegar (1 tablespoon)
- ○ 🍚 Balsamic vinegar (1 tablespoon)
- ○ 🍚 Salsa (18-ounce jar)

Cooking Oils:
- ○ Olive oil ($1/4$ cup)

Pastas and Tomato Products:
- ○ Chopped tomatoes
  (two 19-ounce cans)
- ○ Unsalted tomato paste (6-ounce can)

Canned Beans and Soup Broths:
- ○ Red kidney beans (19-ounce can)

Spices and Seasonings:
- ○ Bay leaf (1)
- ○ Chile powder (2 tablespoons)
- ○ Dried rosemary (1 teaspoon)
- ○ Dried oregano (2 tablespoons)
- ○ Garlic powder (1 teaspoon)

KEY: 🍚 denotes Second Supper or Grab & Go Lunch items

SHOPPING LIST

○ Ground cumin (1 teaspoon)
○ 🍲 Dried thyme (1 teaspoon)

Grains:
○ Quinoa or tiny pasta (1 cup)

Juices:
○ 🍲 Any 100% juice (4 single-serving
boxes)

Notes:

KEY: 🍲 denotes Second Supper or Grab *&* Go Lunch items

WEEK

11

GROWN-UP KIDS
OF ALL AGES

T HE LAST TWO weeks of this book contain more sophisticated recipes for older, more adventurous palates, paying special attention to fish. Adding fish to any diet is an important shift to make for overall health, but especially for the growing brains and bodies of teenagers. There are many schools of thought around fish these days, but the general consensus is that the benefits of fresh or farmed fish still far outweigh the potential negatives of contamination. I suppose you get to choose your poison: the heart-healthy lean protein with omega-3 brain builders now versus the possible effects of toxins later. The best way to handle this issue is to spread out your consumption. Most experts agree that you can eat fish up to three times per week without any harm being done, while reaping huge benefits. Educate yourself about where your fish comes from and try to vary the types you eat. Switch it up a bit from deep ocean fish to lake fish to bivalves and crustaceans. A wide variety ensures that you get good nutrients and reduces the risk of build-up of any one kind of toxin from one area.

Here are my top picks: Salmon, either farmed or wild—enjoy it in moderation for its omega-3 goodness. Shrimp and scallops are a great protein to add right out of the freezer to any pasta sauce or soup. Canned clams make an amazing, lean protein addition to soups. Choose Pacific sole when you are looking for a mild, quick-cooking fish (Atlantic sole is overfished). Rainbow trout is best straight up and fried in butter because it is a tender lake fish with good omega-3 counts. Canned tuna is the perennial favorite for its ease. Lobster (for special occasions only since its mercury levels can be high) is just oh, so good.

WEEK 11 MENU CHART

SERVE	MAIN DISH	SERVE WITH
TONIGHT	Creamy Baked Salmon	Balsamic Barley Salad and mixed greens
2ND NIGHT	Bistro Burgers	French bread croutons and mixed greens
3RD NIGHT	Southwestern Fish Sticks	Guacamole, corn, mixed greens
4TH NIGHT	🍲 Barbecued Meatballs	Roasted Radicchio Salad, tomato sauce
5TH NIGHT	🍲 Fish and Potato Pie	Cucumber and parsley salad
GRAB & GO LUNCH	Barley Salad with Cottage Cheese and Greens	
GRAB & GO LUNCH	Asian Salmon Sandwich	

🍲 = Second Supper recipe

WORK SCHEDULE

1 Simmer barley for Balsamic Barley Salad. Turn off when cooked; complete later.

2 Assemble Southwestern Fish Sticks and freeze.

3 Mix Guacamole and store in freezer.

4 Prepare the salmon and store in fridge until you are aready to prepare supper for tonight.

5 Complete Balsamic Barley Salad and store in fridge, covered, until you are ready to serve tonight.

6 Make the burgers (and meatballs) last to avoid spreading any bacteria from raw meat; freeze. Skip croutons until the day you are serving the burgers.

Balsamic Barley Salad

> **SERVES:** 4 as side dish + 4 as side dish with Barbecued Meatballs
> Second Supper + 2 for Grab & Go Lunch
> **PREPARATION TIME:** 11 minutes

Spend a few *extra dollars on a good bottle of balsamic vinegar. It is much less acidic than the less expensive kind and the difference is noticeable.*

2 to 2½ cups pot barley
3 cups water
2 cups beef stock (preferably frozen or homemade)
1 cup frozen corn niblets
1 cup frozen green beans
1 cup frozen peas
½ cup balsamic vinegar
¼ cup extra-virgin olive oil
2 tablespoons soy sauce
Salt and pepper to taste

◆ In very large pot, bring barley, water, and stock to boil. Reduce heat and simmer for 40 minutes, until barley is chewable. Turn off heat even though there may still be some water left—it will absorb eventually or be mixed in with the dressing.
◆ Break green beans into barley while still warm. Add corn and peas; stir. Add vinegar, oil, soy sauce, salt, and pepper. Cover and let stand until cool. Empty into serving bowl and cover with plastic wrap.

TIPS

NEVER UNDERESTIMATE THE power of the frozen vegetable! It is often more nutritious than its fresh counterpart, which may have traveled and been improperly stored for many days. If you have leftover frozen corn, it is great thawed and mixed with salsa as a dip for corn chips.

Barley Salad with Cottage Cheese and Greens

THERE WILL BE lots of barley salad made with this recipe and it will keep in the fridge for up to 5 days. Serve it with everything. For a nice light lunch packed with complex carbohydrates and protein, and loaded with fiber, line a plate with lettuce and top with a mound of barley salad and a mound of cottage cheese Add some fresh fruit on the side to fill you up.

SERVES: 1 to 3 ➤ **PREPARATION TIME:** 3 minutes

Southwestern Fish Sticks

SERVES: 4 as entrée + 4 for Second Supper
PREPARATION TIME: 20 minutes

Serve these with *plum sauce and Guacamole (page 132) as well as some frozen corn that has been warmed in the microwave or in a pot. The addition of a mixed green salad makes this a light and nourishing meal full of good fats and brain food.*

1 cup yellow cornmeal (see Tips)
²/₃ cup Italian-seasoned bread crumbs
½ cup grated Parmesan cheese
2 tablespoon chile powder
1 tablespoon ground cumin
1 tablespoon garlic powder
1 teaspoon granulated sugar
1 teaspoon hot pepper flakes
½ teaspoon white pepper
2 pounds Pacific cod fillets (or Pacific haddock) (see Tips)
½ cup milk
¼ cup plum sauce (see Tips)

◆ In large zip-top plastic bag, combine cornmeal, bread crumbs, Parmesan, chile powder, cumin, garlic powder, sugar, hot pepper flakes, and white pepper; shake well.
◆ Line with foil a baking sheet small enough to fit into freezer; spray foil with cooking spray.
◆ Rinse fish under cold water; slice into 3 x ½-inch sticks. In another freezer bag, mix plum sauce with milk; add fish and gently toss to coat. Place 3 or 4 fish fingers at a time into cornmeal mixture and shake gently. Place on baking sheet; spray top of each with cooking spray. Freeze, uncovered, for 2 to 4 hours; transfer to zip-top plastic bag. (Can be frozen for up to 3 weeks.)
◆ Preheat oven to 375°F. Place desired number of frozen fish sticks on baking sheet. Bake in 375°F oven for 20 to 35 minutes, until firm and slightly browned.

TIPS

THE COMMON CHINESE plum sauce that kids love to use as dip is usually found in the "ethnic" or "Asian" section of the grocery store or sometimes with the ketchup. Although sweet, it actually has some minor nutrient value. Not from the plums, but from the pumpkin puree that is often added to make the sauce orange. Who knew?

Cornmeal makes an awesome side dish. In the South it's called grits but in Italy it is polenta. Either way, this whole-grain pasta substitute is simple. Simmer 3 parts water with 1 part cornmeal for 15 minutes, stirring often. Add water as needed. Stir in generous amounts of salt and pepper as well as a tablespoon or two of butter at the end of the cooking time, and call it grits. Or press leftovers into a cake or loaf pan to be cut into squares and pan-fried in olive oil, and call it polenta; top it with Parmesan cheese.

I have specified Pacific cod here only because Atlantic cod tends to be overfished and we need to think about our planet as well as our plate.

Fish and Potato Pie

The fish sticks form the foundation of this soft and comforting casserole served with a side of cucumber and parsley salad.

> 5 cups water
> 6 medium-size white new potatoes, scrubbed but not peeled
> 1½ cups parsley
> ¼ cup milk
> 2 tablespoons butter
> Salt and pepper to taste
> 8 to 10 reserved frozen Southwestern Fish Sticks
> 1 cup frozen peas (optional)
> 2 tablespoons Italian-seasoned bread crumbs
> ¼ cup grated Parmesan cheese

SIDE SALAD:
> 2 English cucumbers, washed but not peeled
> 2 tablespoons seasoned rice vinegar
> 2 tablespoons extra-virgin olive oil

◆ Preheat oven to 375°F.

◆ Bring water to a boil while you roughly chop potatoes into 3-inch pieces. Drop potatoes into water, cover, and simmer for 15 minutes, or until potatoes are soft. While potatoes are boiling, immerse parsley in a large bowl of very cold water and swirl to remove sand. Pull parsley from water, leaving sand in the bowl. Empty and rinse the bowl. Use clean kitchen scissors to roughly chop parsley back into the bowl, set aside.

◆ When potatoes are cooked, drain off any remaining water and add milk, butter, and salt and pepper. Mash with a potato masher or handheld blender to desired consistency. Place frozen Southwestern Fish Sticks in the bottom of a casserole dish and top with potatoes. Sprinkle top of potatoes with bread crumbs and Parmesan cheese. Bake, uncovered for 25 to 30 minutes.

◆ Finish side salad while pie is baking. Using the slicing side of a box grater, slice cucumbers directly into the bowl of parsley. Pour vinegar and olive oil over and toss.

SERVES: 4 ➤ **PREPARATION TIME:** 12 to 15 minutes

Guacamole

SERVES: 4 as side dish + 4 for Grab & Go Lunch + 4 as afterschool snacks
PREPARATION TIME: 15 minutes

A**vocados are one** *of my favorite fruits, full of flavor. Although they do contain a measure of fat, it is the healthy kind. Sweet pickle relish plays a minor role in the flavors here and, although it sounds odd, it does add just a hint of a recognizable sweetness to this dip and helps keep it green.*

> 3 green onions, trimmed
> 6 ripe avocados (see Tip)
> 1 tablespoon sweet pickle relish
> 1 teaspoon dried thyme
> 3 tablespoons fresh lime juice
> Cooking spray

- Using handheld blender or mini chopper, finely mince green onions, including fair bit of green parts to keep dip green during freezing.
- Slice avocados in half; squeeze out flesh into bowl. Discard pit and skin. Add relish and thyme to flesh; mash with fork to leave a few chunks or use handheld blender to puree. Add green onions and half of the lime juice; stir.
- Empty into three ramekins or small serving dishes; pour remaining lime juice over tops then spray with oil to prevent browning. Cover tightly with plastic wrap and freeze up to 2 weeks. To serve, remove from freezer at least 2 hours before serving, to thaw. Serve with blue corn tortilla chips, or Southwestern Fish Sticks.

TIP

STORING CUT AVOCADO is tricky because the flesh browns so quickly. If you spray the cut side with cooking spray lightly before wrapping and refrigerating, your avocado should stay green.

Creamy Baked Salmon

> **SERVES:** 4 as entrée + 2 for Grab & Go Lunch
> **PREPARATION TIME:** 15 minutes

*E*vaporated skim milk *makes this dish creamy without adding fat. Serve with some mixed greens and Balsamic Barley Salad (page 127).*

  1½ pounds salmon fillets
  1 teaspoon dried tarragon
  ¼ teaspoon salt
  Pepper to taste
  1 (8-ounce) can evaporated skim milk

◆ Rinse salmon under cold water and pat dry with paper towel. Lay salmon in large, shallow ceramic or glass baking dish. Sprinkle with tarragon, salt, and pepper; pour evaporated milk over top. (Ideally, the dish is large enough that the salmon is only half submerged.) Cover with plastic wrap and refrigerate up to 8 hours.
◆ Preheat oven to 400°F.
◆ Place the salmon in the oven and bake, uncovered, at 400°F for 12 to 15 minutes, basting twice, until fish flakes easily when tested with fork.

Asian Salmon Sandwich

MASH LEFTOVER SALMON and its liquid with 1 teaspoon toasted sesame oil, 1 tablespoon honey mustard, 1 teaspoon soy sauce and ½ teaspoon grated gingerroot. Place on whole wheat burger bun and top with ½ cup grated cabbage. Some extra grated cabbage on the side sprinkled with toasted sesame oil and soy sauce makes for a high-fiber, delicious side dish.

SERVES: 1 to 2 ➤ **PREPARATION TIME:** 4 minutes

TIP
USE TOASTED SESAME oil, not light, to impart a deep, nutty flavor.

Bistro Burgers

SERVES: 4 as entrée + 4 for Second Supper
PREPARATION TIME: 10 minutes

Here's a versatile *mixture of beef and flavorings that can become either burgers or meatballs. I suggest both!*

BURGERS:

4 green onions
2 pounds extra-lean ground beef
½ cup dry Italian-seasoned bread crumbs
2 eggs
2 teaspoon dried thyme
Salt and pepper to taste

2 cups (6 ounces) sliced mushrooms
2 cups red wine or beef stock
8 slices (½ inch thick) whole-grain bread
2 tablespoons Italian herb seasoning
1 (10-ounce) package fresh baby spinach
2 cups (1 pint) cherry tomatoes

◆ Lay out four pieces of foil about 12 inches long.
◆ Burgers: Finely mince green onions; place in large bowl. Add beef, bread crumbs, eggs, thyme, salt, and pepper; mix well with hands. Divide in half. Use one-half to make four 4-inch diameter patties, pressing firmly. Press a dimple with thumb into center of each. Place 2 patties on each piece of foil and wrap loosely; place in zip-top plastic bag and freeze up to 1 month. Use the second half to make meatballs for second supper. You should get sixteen to twenty 1-inch meatballs, which can be placed in the freezer on a cookie sheet until frozen solid, then transferred to a zip-top freezer bag for storage.
◆ Heat nonstick pan with lid. Brown frozen burgers on each side; remove and pat dry with paper towel. Add mushrooms; stir for 6 to 8 minutes. Place burgers on mushrooms; pour in red wine or stock (or combo of both). Cover and simmer 20 minutes, or until meat thermometer inserted sideways registers 160°F.

- Heat broiler. Lay bread on baking sheet; spray bread with cooking spray. Sprinkle with herbs; broil for 1 to 2 minutes each side (watch carefully).
- Top each with burger; pour some wine jus with mushrooms over top. Serve with spinach and cherry tomatoes.

TIPS

TO MAKE QUICK, plain burgers, simply broil for 15 to 20 minutes. The dimple in the patty fills in as meat cooks and shrinks, and prevents the meat from expanding in the middle, causing it to be raw due to thickness.

If you want to omit the bread altogether, add the Italian herbs to the wine just for added flavor.

Barbecue Meatballs with Roasted Radicchio Salad

16 to 20 reserved meatballs
2 tablespoons barbecue sauce
2 heads radicchio
¼ cup balsamic vinegar
Salt and pepper, to taste
2 cups reserved Balsamic Barley Salad

- Place frozen meatballs on baking sheet and bake, uncovered, in preheated 375°F oven for 25 to 35 minutes. Toss with barbecue sauce and bake further 5 to 10 minutes, until completely cooked through.
- To make Roasted Radicchio, rinse and quarter heads of radicchio and lay in a low-sided casserole dish. Sprinkle with balsamic vinegar and salt and pepper. Bake in oven, along with meatballs, covered in foil for 20 minutes. Top with Barley Salad.
- Serve the meatballs and radicchio, making a fun meal of it by passing toothpicks alongside ramekins of your favorite tomato sauce for dipping the meatballs.

SERVES: 4 ➤ PREPARATION TIME: 10 minutes

WEEK
11

SHOPPING LIST

YOU NEED:

Baked goods:
- ○ Whole-grain bread (1 loaf)
- ○ Italian-seasoned bread crumbs (1½ cups)
- ○ 🥣 Whole wheat hamburger buns (8)

Dairy:
- ○ Eggs (2)
- ○ Milk (¾ cup)
- ○ Parmesan cheese, grated (¾ cup)
- ○ 🥣 Cottage cheese (1 cup)
- ○ Butter (1 tablespoon)

Meat and Alternatives:
- ○ Pacific cod fillets (2 pounds)
- ○ Salmon fillets (1½ pounds)
- ○ Extra-lean ground beef (2 pounds)

Produce:
- ○ Mushrooms, sliced (6 ounces)
- ○ Cherry tomatoes (1 pint)
- ○ Baby spinach (10-ounce package)
- ○ Avocados (6)
- ○ Green onions (1 bunch)
- ○ Lime juice (3 tablespoons)
- ○ 🥣 Gingerroot (½ teaspoon)
- ○ 🥣 Yellow bell pepper (1)
- ○ 🥣 Oranges (2)
- ○ 🥣 Mixed greens (10-ounce package)
- ○ 🥣 Grated cabbage (16-ounce package)
- ○ 🥣 Radicchio (2 heads)
- ○ 🥣 Lettuce (1 head)
- ○ 🥣 Yukon gold potatoes (3 medium-size)
- ○ 🥣 Fresh parsley (1½ cups)
- ○ 🥣 English cucumbers (2)

Frozen Foods:
- ○ Frozen green beans (1 cup)
- ○ Frozen corn niblets (2 cups)
- ○ Frozen peas (2 cups)
- ○ Beef stock (2 cups)

CHECK YOUR PANTRY FOR:

Condiments and Dressings:
- ○ Soy sauce (3 tablespoons)
- ○ Sweet pickle relish (1 tablespoon)
- ○ Plum sauce (¼ cup, plus extra for dipping)
- ○ Balsamic vinegar (½ cup)
- ○ 🥣 Barbecue sauce (2 tablespoons)
- ○ 🥣 Honey mustard (1 tablespoon)
- ○ 🥣 Rice vinegar (2 tablespoons)

Cooking Oils:
- ○ Extra-virgin olive oil (¼ cup plus 2 table-spoons)
- ○ Olive oil (2 tablespoons)
- ○ 🥣 Toasted sesame oil (1 tablespoons)
- ○ 🥣 Vegetable cooking spray

Pastas and Tomato Products:
- ○ 🥣 Tomato Sauce (16-ounce jar)

Baking Products:
- ○ Evaporated skim milk (8-ounce can)
- ○ Granulated sugar (1 teaspoon)

Spices and Seasonings:
- ○ Dried thyme (2 tablespoons)
- ○ Garlic powder (1 tablespoon)
- ○ White pepper (½ teaspoon)

KEY: 🥣 denotes Second Supper or Grab & Go Lunch items

○ Dried tarragon (1 teaspoon)
○ Chile powder (2 tablespoons)
○ Hot pepper flakes (1 teaspoon)
○ Italian herb seasoning (2 tablespoons)
○ Ground cumin (1 tablespoon)

Snack Foods:
○ Blue corn tortilla chips (16-ounce package)

Grains:
○ Yellow cornmeal (1 cup)
○ Pot barley (2 to 2$\frac{1}{2}$ cups)

Wine and Beer:
○ Red wine (2 cups)

Notes:

KEY: 🥣 denotes Second Supper or Grab & Go Lunch items

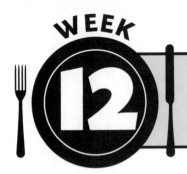

WEEK 12

UNIQUE TASTES

WHETHER I ENTERTAIN two ladies for lunch or an entire family of fussies, I like to sit with my guests. I feel so sad when I see a host slaving over details when her guests really want to catch up with her. What a shame that the cook does all the work and then sits down, exhausted, at 11 PM, when everyone is ready to leave!

Because I do what I do for a living, everyone expects that when they come to my house they will be well fed. This doesn't mean that I do everything myself. Once in a while, I will get the urge to make my own salsa, but most of the time the best bottle I can find will do.

The best advice I can give a host is to plan everything in advance, spend time on the presentation, and cut corners everywhere else. The concept of "good enough" is hard to convey but any one-pot dish served in a soup tureen sprinkled with fresh herbs is pretty easy to do. Homemade biscuits make it special, but you could buy those from a good bakery instead. Roll a cold stick of butter in some chopped herbs, and it looks like you worked all day. Take time with your table and create something unique. Serving salad in lovely little flowerpots makes more of an impression than toiling over the dressing to get the acid balance just right. Use one interesting ingredient, a prickly pear for instance, and you've got dinnertime conversation started.

Best advice I ever got? Never apologize, never explain. If you adhere to this next time you burn the vegetables, your guests will think you invented a new dish: Blackened Green Beans!

MENU 12 CHART

SERVE	MAIN DISH	SERVE WITH
TONIGHT	Scallops and Soybeans in Sake Broth	Rice Crackers
2ND NIGHT	Thai Stuffed Pork with Mashed Apples and Squash	Spicy Asian Salad
3RD NIGHT	Sesame Fish Cakes	Baby Bok Choy
4TH NIGHT	Salad with Roast Pork Loin and Tomatoes	No extras necessary
5TH NIGHT	Easy Fish Chowder	Whole-grain buns
GRAB & GO LUNCH	Pita Stuffed with Pork and Apples	
GRAB & GO LUNCH	Spicy Asian Salad with Soybeans	

 = **Second Supper recipe**

WORK SCHEDULE

1 Start the Sesame Fish Cakes first and let the potatoes cook.

2 Wash and assemble the ingredients for the Scallops and Soybeans in Sake Stock; set on counter or in fridge. Cooking tonight will take only 10 minutes.

3 Make the stuffing for Thai Stuffed Pork; stuff and refrigerate the pork. (Do not prepare Mashed Apples and Squash until the day you are serving.)

4 Make the dressing for the Spicy Asian Salad; toss just before serving.

5 Optional: Clean and dry romaine lettuce to get a head start on the week. Store wrapped in paper towel, then in plastic bag in crisper.

Sesame Fish Cakes
with Baby Bok Choy

SERVES: 4 as entrée + 4 for Second Supper
PREPARATION TIME: 30 minutes

You could use *any mild white fish in this recipe. Try tilapia; it is the mildest, and so far has safe mercury levels as well as a moderate omega-3 count. This species is, at the moment, not overfished. Other options include Pacific sole (Atlantic is overfished), rainbow trout, or Pacific cod.*

> 6 thin-skinned potatoes (Yukon gold, or white)
> 6 frozen white fish fillets (about 1 pound), thawed
> 2 green onions
> ½ cup chopped fresh parsley
> 1 tablespoon grated gingerroot
> 4 cloves garlic, minced
> 1 tablespoon salt

COATING:
> ¼ cup cornmeal
> ¼ cup sesame seeds
> 1 tablespoon curry powder

BABY BOK CHOY:
> 4 baby bok choy
> 2 tablespoons seasoned rice vinegar
> 1 (8-ounce) jar sweet chile sauce

◆ Scrub (but do not peel) potatoes; chop into quarters. In large pot of boiling water, cook potatoes for 15 minutes until soft enough to be poked with knife. Add fish; simmer for 2 to 4 minutes until fish flakes easily when tested with fork.

◆ Meanwhile, rinse green onions under cold running water. Chop, then place in large bowl; add parsley, ginger, garlic, and salt.

◆ Coating: On plate, mix cornmeal, sesame seeds, and curry powder; set aside. Drain fish mixture. (Set aside any children's portions that you wish to keep plain to roll in plain cornmeal and salt, and freeze with the seasoned ones.) Add potatoes and fish to green onion mixture; mash with potato masher or handheld blender until soft but not smooth. Let cool.

- Spray three or four large pieces of foil with cooking spray.
- Form potato mixture by ½ cupfuls into 10 to 12 patties. Roll in cornmeal mixture and place on foil; spray tops with cooking spray and fold foil over. Freeze up to 3 weeks (reserve 4 fish patties for Easy Fish Chowder Second Supper, below).
- Spray large skillet with cooking spray; heat over medium-high heat. Brown 3 or 4 patties at a time on one side before turning carefully. Cover to allow to warm through, turning once more. Reduce heat to medium-low.
- Meanwhile, pull leaves of baby bok choy apart and rinse. Place in large microwavable bowl; sprinkle with rice vinegar, and toss with sweet chile sauce. Cover and microwave on high for 4 to 6 minutes, just to soften. (Or steam in a large, low pot with 1 inch of boiling water for 4 to 6 minutes. Drain and toss with rice vinegar and sweet chile sauce. Serve with fish cakes.

Easy Fish Chowder

I always say that a slow cooker is a family's best friend, but this recipe can be made easily on the stovetop as well.

> 4 reserved frozen Sesame Fish Cakes
> 4 to 6 cups frozen chicken broth, or low-salt canned
> 2 cups frozen corn niblets
> 1 (16-ounce) can baby clams
> 4 tablespoons whipping cream
> 1 tablespoon sherry
> 1 (10-ounce) package prewashed mixed greens
> Salad dressing, for serving greens

- Slow-cooker method: Place frozen fish cakes in slow cooker; add chicken stock. Cook on low for 3 to 4 hours; stir well to be sure it is well mixed. Add frozen corn and baby clams, undrained. Turn slow cooker up to high, let cook for 30 to 40 minutes just to warm through. Stir in the cream; drizzle with sherry. Serve with mixed greens and your favorite dressing alongside.
- Stovetop method: Bring chicken broth to a boil over high heat and add frozen fish cakes to warm through and break up, about 20 minutes. Stir in corn and baby clams, undrained, and simmer for 5 more minutes. Stir in the cream; drizzle with sherry. Serve with mixed greens and your favorite dressing alongside.

SERVES: 4 ➤ PREPARATION TIME: 8 to 10 minutes

Scallops and Soybeans in Sake Stock

SERVES: 4
PREPARATION TIME: 10 minutes

This is a *very light meal, great for hot evenings when you don't feel like making a big fuss. Serve in large pasta bowls with rice crackers on the side.*

  2 tablespoon olive oil
  1 (4-ounce) package frozen scallops, thawed
  2 cups sake, or 1 cup white wine
  2 cups chicken stock (preferably homemade or frozen)
  2 cups frozen soybeans (edamame), shelled (see Tips)
  1 tablespoon chile sauce
  ½ pound broccoli rabe, well rinsed and trimmed, or broccoli florets (see Tips)

◆ In large ovenproof skillet, heat oil. Brown scallops slightly, about 2 minutes per side, then flip. (At this point if you like you can remove any children's portions and try serving them with raw or steamed broccoli and a small cup of broth on the side.) Cover the scallops with foil and let stand on stove to keep warm and continue cooking.

◆ Preheat broiler. Pour sake and chicken stock over scallops; bring to boil. Simmer for 5 minutes. Add soybeans and chile sauce. Lay the broccoli rabe over the scallops and baste with liquid. Place entire skillet on broiler rack 4 inches from heat; broil for 2 to 6 minutes, until warmed through.

TIPS

FROZEN SOYBEANS ARE a great source of protein and are simple to prepare. If you can purchase the already-shelled beans, all they need to make a great snack or side dish is a quick steaming for 4 to 5 minutes and a sprinkling of some salt or soy sauce.

Broccoli rabe is the bitter cousin of broccoli, not because it gets chosen less often but because its flavor is much stronger. All it needs is a quick steaming on the stovetop or in the microwave. Try chopping it into smaller pieces and sprinkling with sugar, balsamic vinegar, olive oil, and Parmesan cheese. This Italian vegetable can hold its own served with any hearty meat, like ribs or beef.

Thai Stuffed Pork with Mashed Apples and Squash

> **SERVES:** 4 as entrée + 4 for Second Supper + 2 for Grab & Go Lunch
> **PREPARATION TIME:** 18 minutes

The peanuty flavors and fresh basil used in this pork are reminiscent of Thai cuisine. The mashed apples and squash are a snap to make.

2 cups matzo meal or crushed crackers
½ cup bottled peanut sauce
¼ cup water
1 tablespoon toasted sesame oil
1 teaspoon aniseed
2 cloves garlic, minced
4 (1-pound) pork tenderloins, butterflied
1 bunch fresh basil, rinsed, drained, and stemmed
¼ cup balsamic vinegar
2 red bell peppers, seeded, cored, and sliced

MASHED APPLES AND SQUASH:
2 cups frozen apple slices
2 cups frozen squash
2 tablespoons butter
½ teaspoon nutmeg

◆ Mix together matzo meal, peanut sauce, water, sesame oil, aniseed, and garlic for stuffing.

◆ Lay out two large pieces of foil. Cut four pieces of butcher's twine. Lay a butterflied tenderloin on foil; top with half of the stuffing, top with half of the basil. Place second butterflied tenderloin on top. Slide two pieces of twine under bottom and tie the tenderloin into thirds widthwise. Drizzle with balsamic vinegar, spray with cooking spray, and wrap in foil. Repeat with other tenderloins. Freeze in zip-top plastic bags for up to 4 weeks. Thaw in refrigerator overnight if you will be serving twice as is or baking both together to use as a Second Supper.

◆ Preheat oven to 325°F. Place pork on baking sheet with foil opened flat; arrange red peppers around pork. Bake in 325°F oven for 1 hour, until stuffing is hot and juices run clear when pork is pierced. Cut and gently remove strings, and slice pork diagonally to keep layers intact. (Set aside slices from one set of tenderloins for use in Pork and Tomato Salad Second Supper.)

◆ Mashed Apples and Squash: Meanwhile, in microwavable bowl, mix apples, squash, and ¼ cup water; microwave on high for 15 minutes. (Or to cook on stovetop, place sliced apples, squash, and ¼ cup water in a pot and cook over low heat, covered, for 20 minutes or so, watching carefully and stirring often. Mash until chunky but smooth. Add butter and nutmeg. Serve with pork.

Spicy Asian Salad

SERVES: 4 as side dish + 2 for Grab & Go Lunch
PREPARATION TIME: 4 minutes

If you have *a mini chopper or mini food processor, you can make the dressing in half the time.*

1 clove garlic, minced
½ jalapeño pepper, minced
¼ cup firmly packed brown sugar
¼ cup lime juice
¼ cup coconut milk
Salt and pepper to taste
1 (10-ounce) package prewashed mixed greens
¼ cup chopped peanuts

◆ In jar with a tight-fitting lid, shake garlic, jalapeño pepper, brown sugar, lime juice, and coconut milk. Add salt and pepper to taste. (Dressing can be stored in fridge up to 1 week.)

◆ Just before serving, toss greens with dressing and top with peanuts. (Reserve 4 to 6 tablespoons dressing for Second Supper and Grab & Go Lunch, if desired.)

Salad with Roast Pork Loin and Tomatoes

1 reserved stuffed and cooked pork roast, sliced
4 tablespoons dressing from Spicy Asian Salad (page 144)
1 pint cherry tomatoes
Salt and pepper to taste
1 head romaine lettuce, cleaned and torn

DRIZZLE PORK WITH Spicy Asian Salad Dressing and warm in microwave on medium setting for 4 to 6 minutes just to reheat. (Alternatively, warm pork with dressing over medium-low heat on stovetop, covered, for 5 to minutes.) Slice cherry tomatoes in half and toss together with salt and pepper to taste. Serve hot pork and tomatoes over a bed of cold romaine. This recipe can also be served cold on a hot summer night.

SERVES: 4 ➤ **PREPARATION TIME:** 7 minutes

Spicy Asian Salad with Soybeans

PLACE ½ CUP frozen soybeans in a microwave-safe bowl. Sprinkle the beans lightly with soy sauce and microwave on high for 2 to 4 minutes. (Alternatively, place the soybeans in a pot filled with 1 inch of boiling water until defrosted. Drain and toss with a bit of soy sauce.) Pour 1 to 2 tablespoons of Spicy Asian Dressing over beans and toss to combine. Pack bean salad with 2 to 3 cups of mixed greens and top with peanuts. On the side, include some rice crackers, a small container of yogurt, and a banana.

SERVES: 1 to 2 ➤ **PREPARATION TIME:** 4 minutes

YOU NEED:

Baked goods:
- ○ Whole wheat buns (4)

Dairy:
- ○ Butter (2 tablespoons)
- ○ Whipping cream (¼ cup) (optional)
- ○ Yogurt (4 single-serving tubs)

Meat and Alternatives:
- ○ Pork tenderloins (four 1-pound)

Produce:
- ○ Gingerroot (1 tablespoon)
- ○ Thin-skinned potatoes, Yukon gold or white (6)
- ○ Fresh basil (1 bunch)
- ○ Fresh parsley (½ cup)
- ○ Broccoli rabe or broccoli (½ pound)
- ○ Baby bok choy (4)
- ○ Red bell peppers (2)
- ○ Garlic (7 cloves)
- ○ Green onions (2)
- ○ Jalapeño pepper (½)
- ○ Lime juice (¼ cup)
- ○ Cherry tomatoes (1 pint)
- ○ Mixed greens (two 10-ounce packages)
- ○ Romaine lettuce (1 head)
- ○ Red grapes (3 cups)
- ○ Bananas (4)

Frozen Foods:
- ○ Frozen scallops (14-ounce package)
- ○ Frozen white fish fillets, sole, or haddock (1 pound)
- ○ Frozen soybeans (edamame) (2 cups)
- ○ Frozen apple slices (2 cups)
- ○ Frozen squash (2 cups)
- ○ Chicken broth (6 to 8 cups)
- ○ Frozen corn niblets (2 cups)

CHECK YOUR PANTRY FOR:

Condiments and Dressings:
- ○ Sweet chile sauce (8-ounce jar)
- ○ Peanut sauce (½ cup)
- ○ Balsamic vinegar (¼ cup)
- ○ Seasoned rice vinegar (2 tablespoons)

Cooking Oils:
- ○ Olive oil (2 tablespoons)
- ○ Toasted sesame oil (1 tablespoon)

Canned:
- ○ Baby clams (16-ounce can)

Baking Products:
- ○ Brown sugar (¼ cup)

Spices and Seasonings:
- ○ Sesame seeds (¼ cup)
- ○ Curry powder (1 tablespoon)
- ○ Aniseed (1 teaspoon)
- ○ Ground nutmeg (½ teaspoon)
- ○ Coconut milk (¼ cup)

Snack Foods:
- ○ Rice crackers (8 to 12 ounce package)
- ○ Peanuts (¼ cup)

Grains:
- ○ Cornmeal (¼ cup)
- ○ Matzo meal (2 cups)

Wine and Beer:
- ○ Sake (2 cups), or white wine (1 cup)
- ○ Sherry (1 tablespoon) (optional)

KEY: denotes Second Supper or Grab & Go Lunch items

Notes:

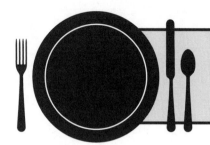

THIS WEEK'S OFFERINGS are intended to make even the pickiest kids happy, and are a great way to ease you and your family into the *Cook Once a Week* system. This week provides the family with a chance to work together on a few of the simplest recipes. I have also included a handful of quick, kid-friendly weeknight recipes that can be pulled together in a snap.

When my daughter was just five weeks old, I met a group of gals who would shape my life forever. The women who met every Friday for fitness and a coffee hour were mothers who had done this all before and had lots to share. I found that they were lawyers, singers, actors, docents, nurses, psychologists, and others who were awe inspiring in many ways. And yet, they were all baffled about how to get meals on the table. That was the one thing I could do! They were the catalyst for my personal chef business.

In the early days, my friend Mary, up the street with little ones, would often call and say, "Let's pool our resources." It was code for, "My husband is working late and the kids are climbing the walls, you too?" We would gather and while away the "witching hours" between 5 and 7 PM.

Making that time go more smoothly, with healthier offerings, is what this week's menus will do. I haven't met anyone who feels good about serving frozen nuggets to her kids. A few recipes like the Homemade Chicken Fingers in your freezer makes suppertime survival a lot easier (and even better when enjoyed with a friend).

BONUS KIDS WEEK MENU CHART

SERVE	MAIN DISH	SERVE WITH
TONIGHT	Lasagne Roll-Ups	Cucumber Faces
2ND NIGHT	Boston Baked Beans	Crudités (see page 47), sliced avocado, and low-fat corn chips
3RD NIGHT	Homemade Chicken Fingers	Mixed greens
4TH NIGHT	Make-Your-Own Pizza Night	No extras necessary
5TH NIGHT	Penne Straws and Peas	No extras necessary
GRAB & GO LUNCH	Grilled Cheese Options	

= Second Supper recipe

WORK SCHEDULE

1 Cook and cool pasta for Lasagne Roll-Ups and then demonstrate assembly to kids—let them continue while you move on to the Boston Baked Beans.

2 Start Boston Baked Beans to bake for the entire day.

3 Lay Lasagne Roll-Ups in pan; cover with cheese, wrap, and refrigerate.

4 Have children combine the bread crumb mixture for the Homemade Chicken Fingers while you rinse and prepare the raw chicken. Then place the chicken in zip-top bags with the bread crumb mixture, seal, and let the kids shake the chicken pieces to coat. Remove from the bag and freeze in a single layer on a cookie sheet. Once frozen, you can remove to a clean zip-top freezer bag and store for up to 3 weeks.

5 Have kids wash their hands thoroughly, then assemble the Cucumber Faces.

6 Clean and chop veggies so you'll have crudités throughout the week.

7 The recipes for Make Your Own Pizza Night and Penne Straws and Peas are a departure from the rest of the book in that they are intended to be made on the night that they are served. These last-minute supper ideas will fill in the week with some simple all-time favorites.

Lasagne Roll-Ups

SERVES: 4 as entrée + 2 for Grab & Go Lunch
PREPARATION TIME: 15 minutes

This is the *faster way to a fun food.*

> 1 teaspoon canola oil
> 8 spinach lasagna noodles
> 2 teaspoons olive oil
> 1 (8-ounce) package vegetarian ground meat substitute (see Tip)
> 1 (19-ounce) can tomato sauce
> 8 ounces mozzarella cheese, shredded
> 2 teaspoons dried oregano or basil (optional)

◆ Bring large pot of water to boil; add canola oil. Immerse lasagna noodles in water; boil until just softened but not sticky, 10 to 12 minutes. Drain and lay out flat on clean counter or plastic wrap.

◆ Meanwhile, oil large lasagne pan with olive oil and set aside. In large bowl, mix vegetarian ground meat with tomato sauce. Spread some onto each lasagna noodle; top with small amount of cheese. Roll up and place seam-side down in oiled pan. Once the pan is filled with roll-ups, you can top them with more sauce and cheese. Sprinkle with oregano if desired. (Cover and refrigerate up to 2 days.)

◆ Preheat oven to 350°F. Bake roll-ups in oven for 20 minutes. (Let cool, cover, and refrigerate up to 2 days.) To serve as Grab & Go Lunch, reheat the roll-ups as needed in microwave or warm in preheated 350°F oven for 2 to 3 minutes, or until heated through.

TIPS

VEGETARIAN GROUND MEAT substitute is a great ingredient not just for its nutritional value (it's made from soy flour) but also for its ease of use. It needs no browning before adding, so it can be tossed at any point into many recipes. Should you have leftovers or extra packages of it, try sprinkling it on pizza. It will look like ground beef and add protein to this family staple.

Boston Baked Beans

SERVES: 4 as entrée + 4 for Second Supper
PREPARATION TIME: 15 minutes

Serve with a *few low-fat corn chips, some slices of avocado, and crudités for a "cowboy supper."*

4 slices bacon
2 cups chopped onion
1 pound dried navy beans (see Tips)
8 cups water
$\frac{1}{2}$ cup light molasses, plus 1 teaspoon more as needed
2 tablespoons brown mustard
Salt and pepper to taste
1 teaspoon cider vinegar, plus 1 teaspoon more as needed
1 avocado, peeled, pitted, and sliced
Low-fat corn chips, for serving
Crudités (see page 47), for serving

◆ Using large, heavy pot with tight-fitting lid, cook bacon over medium heat for about 7 minutes, until browned and fat is released. Add onion; cook, stirring often, for about 8 minutes. Preheat oven to 300°F.

◆ Meanwhile, rinse beans in colander; remove any discolored beans or pebbles. Add to pot along with water, molasses, mustard, salt, and pepper. Bring to boil and stir for about 10 minutes. Cover and bake in bottom third of 300°F oven for 6 hours, until softened. (Or cook in slow cooker on high for 6 to 8 hours.) Uncover and bake for 1½ hours longer or until sauce thickens, stirring occasionally. If desired, stir in an extra teaspoon each of molasses and vinegar to balance flavors. (Freeze in small serving sizes.) Reheat leftovers in microwave or on the stovetop as needed for Second Supper, and serve with any leftover chips and some salsa.

TIPS

HAVE CHILDREN RINSE beans in a colander and look for any small rocks or pebbles. Anyone who finds one wins a taste of sweet molasses right off of the spoon.

This recipe is a hit for kids when they find out that they are guaranteed to be musical within a few hours of eating. Boys especially find these things very funny!

Homemade Chicken Fingers

SERVES: 4 as entrée + 8 for Second Supper
PREPARATION TIME: 14 minutes

This **bread crumb** *mixture is sufficient to coat 8 pounds of chicken, but we are only preparing 2 pounds, so the extra coating can be stored for future use. Serve the chicken fingers with crudités and salsa as a dip, to get extra veggies in.*

> 4 cups dry whole wheat bread crumbs
> 1 cup cornmeal
> 1 tablespoon paprika
> 2 teaspoons celery salt
> 2 teaspoons onion salt
> 2 teaspoons poultry seasoning
> 1 teaspoon white pepper
> 1 teaspoon dried basil
> ½ teaspoon garlic powder
> ½ cup canola oil
> 2 pounds boneless skinless chicken breasts (see Tips)
> Crudités (see page 47), for serving
> Mild salsa, for serving

◆ In large bowl, stir together bread crumbs, cornmeal, paprika, celery salt, onion salt, poultry seasoning, pepper, basil, and garlic powder. Add oil and mix again. Divide among four large zip-top plastic bags; freeze three for up to 3 months. Use one for this recipe.
◆ Preheat oven to 350°F. Pat chicken dry with paper towels. Cut each breast lengthwise into three or four strips. Add strips, two at a time, to one of the bags; shake until evenly coated. Lay on baking sheet sprayed with vegetable oil spray. (Freeze until solid; transfer to freezer bags and freeze for up to 3 weeks. Bake, frozen, in preheated 325°F oven for 20 to 30 minutes. For Second Supper, try serving with plum sauce for dipping.)
◆ Bake in 350°F oven for 10 to 15 minutes, or until no longer pink inside.

IF CHICKEN TENDERS are available at your grocery store, buy them. They eliminate the need for slicing the breast and also provide a softer texture that most kids prefer.

These fingers use a fraction of the fat and salt of store-bought chicken fingers. Since they are baked rather than deep-fried in hydrogenated oils like most commercial products, there is no trans-fat. The addition of cornmeal gives the fingers crunch but also adds fiber and extra whole grain to the diet.

Once cooked, these fingers can be refrozen and sent for lunches or on picnics. By lunchtime they thaw to a perfect temperature for eating cold.

Cucumber Faces

SERVES: 4 as side dish + 4 for Grab & Go Lunch
PREPARATION TIME: 2 minutes

This is a *great side dish and afterschool snack as well as an art activity—how can you go wrong?*

2 English cucumbers (see Tip)
2 carrots
½ cup light cream cheese

◆ Slice cucumbers into rounds. Grate carrots into bowl.
◆ Spread cream cheese onto cucumber rounds. Allow each child to make as many funny faces as possible by sticking on strips of carrot for eyes, nose, and mouth. Use immediately, or cover and refrigeratefor up to 8 hours. For an at-home lunch, serve Cucumber Faces, or the fixin's for them, alongside a hearty sandwich.

TIP

MOST KIDS WILL eat cucumbers although they are not the most nutritious vegetable. So we start showing our commitment to vegetables by making this one fun. We use English cucumbers because their skins are thin enough to be washed and eaten. The waxy kind are not good for this, and provide even fewer vitamins.

Make-Your-Own Pizza Night

SERVES: 4 as entrée
PREPARATION TIME: 5 to 6 minutes

This is a *quick weeknight meal that you can make from what you have on hand—like whole wheat pitas, shredded mozzarella cheese, smoked turkey, tomato paste—anything goes. (All of the items listed below are included in this week's shopping list.)*

> 4 whole wheat pitas
> 5 ounces tomato paste
> 8 ounces low-fat mozzarella cheese, shredded
> 4 slices smoked turkey
> 6 ounces mushrooms, sliced
> Dash of each: garlic powder, dried oregano, dried basil
> 4 tablespoons wheat germ

◆ Preheat oven to 400°F. Place everything on the table and let everyone build an individual pizza. Begin by coating the pita bread with tomato paste, but leaving a ½-inch edge all around for the crust. Divide the cheese, turkey, and mushrooms among the pizzas. Supervise the sprinkling of garlic powder, oregano and basil. Top everyone's pizza with wheat germ to add much needed fiber as well as healthy fats. Bake in 400°F for 10 to 15 minutes on a cookie sheet.

Penne Straws and Peas

SERVES: 4 as entrée
PREPARATION TIME: 3 minutes

Most kids like *tomato sauce, so we are always looking for ways to get other good nutrition into it.*

1 (24-ounce) can tomato sauce
6 ounces vegetarian ground meat substitute
4 cups whole wheat penne
2 cups frozen baby peas
½ cup grated Parmesan cheese

- Empty can of tomato sauce into a pot while you boil water for pasta in another. Add vegetarian ground meat substitute to the tomato sauce and warm through.
- When water boils add penne and cook until almost al dente. Add frozen peas to the pasta water for the final 2 minutes.
- Drain pasta and peas and toss with sauce; top with Parmesan.

Grilled Cheese Options

etting kids to make their own meals as early as possible is a huge bonus not only for the chief cook but also for the self-esteem of the little ones. Sandwich presses are a great way to get kids started. Serve with crudités.

2 ounces butter
8 slices whole-grain bread
4 slices white Cheddar and/or Swiss cheese
4 slices ham or smoked turkey
Ketchup, for dipping (for kids)
Mango chutney, for dipping (for adults)
Crudités (see page 47), for serving

Simply lay out the butter, bread, sliced cheese, ham, smoked turkey, and some ketchup and chutney. Let the kids build their own sandwiches, spreading the butter on the outside of the bread and chosen fillings on the inside. Place sandwiches in the grilling machine or in a skillet over medium-high heat for 3 to 5 minutes per side until outsides are browned and insides begin to melt. Adults may like the grown-up flavor of white Cheddar with a teaspoon of mango chutney in their grilled cheese. Be sure to help those under twelve, since both skillets and sandwich presses can get hot.

SERVES: 4 ➤ PREPARATION TIME: 18 to 20 minutes

TIPS

ONCE KIDS GET the hang of using a sandwich press, they can experiment with dessert sandwich grills. Try apple pie filling and Brie, peanut butter and jam, or pumpkin pie filling.

YOU NEED:

Baked goods:
- ☐ Whole wheat bread crumbs (4 cups)
- ☐ Whole wheat pita (4)
- ☐ Whole-grain bread (8 slices)

Dairy:
- ☐ Light cream cheese (½ cup)
- ☐ Mozzarella cheese, shredded (1 pound)
- ☐ Parmesan cheese, grated (½ cup)
- ☐ 🥣 White Cheddar and/or Swiss cheese (4 slices)
- ☐ 🥣 Butter (2 ounces)
- ☐ 🥣 Brie (5 ounces) (optional)

Meat and Alternatives:
- ☐ Bacon (4 slices)
- ☐ Boneless skinless chicken breasts (2 pounds)
- ☐ Vegetarian ground meat substitute (6- to 8-ounce package)
- ☐ 🥣 Smoked Turkey (4 slices)
- ☐ 🥣 Smoked Ham (4 slices)

Produce:
- ☐ Onions (2)
- ☐ English cucumbers (2)
- ☐ Avocados (2)
- ☐ Celery (1 head)
- ☐ Baby carrots (2 lb)
- ☐ Yellow bell peppers (2)
- ☐ Green Beans (4 cups)
- ☐ Baby spinach (8-ounce package)
- ☐ Mushrooms, sliced (6 ounces)

Frozen Foods:
- ☐ Frozen peas (2 cups)

CHECK YOUR PANTRY FOR:

Condiments and Dressings:
- ☐ Brown mustard (2 tablespoons)
- ☐ Cider vinegar (2 teaspoons)
- ☐ Plum sauce (¼ cup)
- ☐ 🥣 Ketchup (¼ cup)
- ☐ 🥣 Mango chutney (½ cup)
- ☐ Peanut butter (1 jar) (optional)

Cooking Oils:
- ☐ Canola oil (½ cup plus 1 teaspoon)
- ☐ Olive oil (2 teaspoons)

Pastas and Tomato Products:
- ☐ Spinach lasagna noodles (1 pound, about 8 noodles)
- ☐ Tomato sauce (19-ounce can and 24-ounce can)
- ☐ Salsa (18-ounce jar)
- ☐ 🥣 Tomato paste (5 ounces)
- ☐ Whole wheat penne (4 cups)

Baking Products:
- ☐ Light molasses (½ cup)
- ☐ 🥣 Apple pie filling (21-ounce can) (optional)
- ☐ 🥣 Pumpkin Pie Filling (15-ounce can) (optional)

Spices and Seasonings:
- ☐ Poultry seasoning (2 teaspoons)
- ☐ Dried basil (3 teaspoons)
- ☐ Dried oregano (4 teaspoons)
- ☐ White pepper (1 teaspoon)
- ☐ Garlic powder (½ teaspoon)
- ☐ Celery salt (2 teaspoons)
- ☐ Paprika (1 tablespoon)

KEY: 🥣 denotes Second Supper or Grab & Go Lunch items

○ Onion salt (2 teaspoon)

Snack Foods:

○ Low-fat corn chips (16-ounce package)

○ Jam (1 cup) (optional)

Grains:

○ Dried navy beans (1 pound)

○ Cornmeal (1 cup)

○ Wheat germ (4 tablespoons)

Wine and Beer:

○ Red Wine (for drinking!) (optional)

Notes:

KEY: 🥣 denotes Second Supper or Grab & Go Lunch items

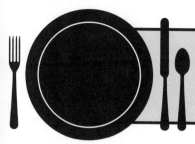

DESSERTS AND SNACKS

I BELIEVE THAT every mouthful should have some nutritional value, but this doesn't mean we can't have a treat now and then. All of the desserts here have at least one thing going for them: they might contain a fruit or a vegetable, protein in the form of nuts, whole grains, or perhaps a little of each. You will not find one drop of trans-fat. You will find only real butter, whole eggs, and a bit of sugar.

Many of these desserts and snacks are just fine to be served as breakfast. Sugary cereals contain minimal amounts of protein, minerals, and vitamins for their calories, but our desserts, containing good things like sweet potatoes, pumpkin, and zucchini, are nutritionally dense in comparison. Best of all, they're fun to eat and easy to make.

Crisp Topping

Pumpkin Pie

Sweet Potato Muffins

Zucchini Muffins

Oh Mega Crackers

Oatmeal Cookies

Quick and Delicious Peanut Butter Cookies

Whole Wheat Graham Crackers

Chewy Biscotti

Banana Boats

Granola Bars

Q-Bix

Sticky Rice Pudding

Vanilla Almond Shake

Crisp Topping

SERVES: 12

PREPARATION TIME: 10 minutes

Yes, **there is** *butter and sugar in this topping but there are also oats and almonds, so the key will be portion size. Kids can eat this by the handful like a granola but the best way to serve it is with warm fruit (see Tip).*

> ¼ **cup whole wheat flour**
> 1 **cup packed brown sugar**
> 1 **cup rolled oats**
> 1 **cup slivered almonds**
> 1 **teaspoon ground cinnamon**
> ¼ **teaspoon grated nutmeg**
> ½ **cup butter, melted**

◆ Preheat oven to 375°F. In bowl, combine flour, sugar, oats, nuts, cinnamon, and nutmeg; blend in butter until crumbly. Spread on baking sheet. Bake in top third of 375°F oven for 18 to 20 minutes, until browned and crispy. Let cool completely. Refrigerate in jar or zip-top plastic bag for up to 3 weeks.

TIP

Choose any frozen fruit you desire; we like apples or blueberries. Microwave a bowl of frozen fruit until melted and warmed. Top with a spoonful or two of the topping. A dollop of low-fat vanilla yogurt makes it even better. You can also use this to top ice cream or sliced berries. A little goes a long way.

Pumpkin Pie

SERVES: 6
PREPARATION TIME: 10 minutes

Ît is the *crust that makes pumpkin pie so decadent, but the truth is that pumpkin is a very nutritious vegetable. If we can garner all of the good and dispense with the bad, we can serve dessert every night!*

> 1 (28-ounce) can pure pumpkin
> ³/₄ cup evaporated skim milk
> 2 eggs
> ½ cup packed brown sugar
> 2 tablespoons pumpkin pie spice
> ¼ teaspoon cream of tartar

◆ Preheat oven to 350°F. Butter and flour pie plate; set aside. In bowl, mix together pumpkin, evaporated milk, eggs, sugar, pumpkin pie spice, and cream of tartar; pour into prepared pie plate. Bake in 350°F oven for 1 hour, or until firm.

Sweet Potato Muffins

SERVES: 12
PREPARATION TIME: 30 minutes

Freeze, wrapped individually, *for lunches or snacks. Serve for dessert or warm in oven for breakfast.*

½ cup butter, softened
1 cup packed brown sugar
1½ cups mashed cooked sweet potatoes
1 egg
¾ cup whole wheat flour
¾ cup all-purpose flour
2 teaspoons pumpkin pie spice
1 teaspoon baking soda
⅓ cup milk to thin butter

◆ Preheat oven to 375°F. In bowl and using electric mixer, cream butter and brown sugar together until fluffy. Beat in sweet potatoes and egg.

◆ Sift together whole wheat and all-purpose flours, pumpkin pie spice, and baking soda. Mix half into sweet potato mixture. Add only enough milk to thin batter. Add remaining dry ingredients. Add enough of the milk to make very thick batter.

◆ Butter and flour muffin pan or use paper liners. Fill muffin cups two-thirds full. Bake in 375°F oven until dry on top and fork comes out clean, 15 to 22 minutes. Let cool. Wrap individually and freeze.

TIP

IF YOU HAVE leftover sweet potatoes, they are the best to use (just remove and discard the skin). If not, pierce 2 medium-size sweet potatoes with a fork, microwave on high for 10 to 20 minutes until cooked. Let cool, then peel and mash them.

Zucchini Muffins

SERVES: 24

PREPARATION TIME: 30 minutes

When your neighbor's *garden overgrows huge zucchini onto your side of the fence, you now have a solution.*

    3 eggs
    1²/₃ cups granulated sugar
    ½ cup canola oil
    ¼ cup butter, softened
    ¼ cup almond butter
    1½ teaspoons vanilla extract
    1½ cups all-purpose flour
    1½ cups whole wheat flour
    2 teaspoons ground cinnamon
    1 teaspoon baking powder
    1 teaspoon baking soda
    1 teaspoon salt
    1 teaspoon grated nutmeg
    3 cups coarsely shredded zucchini
    1 cup seedless raisins (optional)
    2 tablespoons ground flaxseed

◆ Preheat oven to 350°F. In bowl, beat eggs until light with whisk or electric mixers. Gradually add sugar, oil, butter, then almond butter and vanilla extract.

◆ In separate bowl and using fork, mix together all-purpose and whole wheat flours, cinnamon, baking powder, baking soda, salt, and nutmeg. Stir in zucchini. Add to sugar mixture and beat until smooth. Stir in raisins if desired, and flaxseed.

◆ Spoon into nonstick or paper-lined muffin cups until three-quarters full. Bake in 350°F oven 12 to 15 minutes for mini muffins, 15 to 20 for full size. Let cool. Freeze and warm for 15 seconds in microwave oven.

Oh Mega Crackers

SERVES: 18
PREPARATION TIME: 15 minutes

These are named *for their high omega-3 content derived from nuts and wheat germ.*

3 tablespoons wheat germ
1 teaspoon packed brown sugar
1 teaspoon dry yeast
^{1}/₃ cup warm water (105° to 115°F)
^{1}/₄ cup ground almonds
1 tablespoon ground flaxseed
1 tablespoon olive oil
1 teaspoon salt
^{3}/₄ cup whole wheat flour
2 to 3 tablespoons all-purpose flour, for rolling out
1 teaspoon onion salt
1 teaspoon garlic powder
1 teaspoon chile powder

◆ Preheat oven to 350°F. Spread wheat germ on baking sheet; bake in 350°F oven for 10 minutes, stirring after 5 minutes. Set aside, and turn off oven.

◆ In large bowl, dissolve brown sugar and yeast in warm water; let stand 5 minutes. Add wheat germ, almonds, flaxseed, oil and salt; stir well. Stir in whole wheat flour to form stiff dough. Turn out onto lightly floured surface. Knead until smooth and elastic, about 10 minutes, sprinkling with only enough all-purpose flour, 1 tablespoon at a time, to prevent dough from sticking to hands. Place in bowl coated with cooking spray, turning to coat top. Cover and let rise in warm (85°) draft-free place until doubled in bulk, about 1 hour.

◆ Preheat oven to 350°F. Punch dough down. Roll into 10½ × 9-inch paper-thin rectangle on baking sheet coated with cooking spray. Score by making lengthwise and crosswise cuts to form eighteen crackers. Prick surface liberally with fork. Sprinkle with onion salt, garlic powder, and chile powder.

◆ Bake in 350°F oven for 15 minutes, or until browned and crisp. Remove from pan; let cool completely on wire rack. Separate into crackers and store in airtight container.

Oatmeal Cookies

MAKES: 60   SERVES: 30
PREPARATION TIME: 15 minutes

*K*eep a close *eye on these cookies as they bake: 8 to 10 minutes will make them soft but 10 to 12 will make them crispy. If you want chewier cookies, place the dough on the cookie sheet in small balls, which will flatten during baking. If you like your cookies crispy, press the dough mounds slightly flat before you bake them.*

1 cup butter
2 cups all-purpose flour
1 teaspoon ground cinnamon
1 teaspoon baking soda
1 teaspoon baking powder
1 cup packed brown sugar
1 cup granulated sugar
2 eggs, beaten lightly
3 cups rolled oats
½ cup seedless raisins

◆ Preheat oven to 350°F. Melt butter and cool to room temperature; place in large bowl.
◆ In separate bowl, sift together flour, cinnamon, baking soda, and baking powder.
◆ Add brown and granulated sugars to butter and stir well. Add eggs, sifted dry ingredients, oats, and raisins. Drop by tablespoonfuls onto well-greased baking sheets.
◆ Bake in 350°F oven for 8 to 12 minutes, depending on desired crispness.

Quick and Delicious
Peanut Butter Cookies

MAKES: 24   **SERVES:** 12
PREPARATION TIME: 30 minutes

You can feel *okay about serving these for breakfast. They are a good source of protein, served with a glass of milk.*

1 cup peanut butter (natural, unsweetened, without hydrogenated oils)
²/₃ cup granulated sugar
1 egg
1 teaspoon all-purpose flour

◆ Preheat oven to 350°F. In bowl, combine peanut butter, sugar, and egg; blend well. Sprinkle with flour to make balls easier to shape.
◆ Form into twenty-four 1-inch balls. Place 1½ to 2 inches apart on greased baking sheets. Using fork, press crisscross pattern into dough.
◆ Bake in 350°F oven 12 to 15 minutes, or until lightly browned. Cool on wire rack.

Whole Wheat Graham Crackers

MAKES: 12 to 18   **SERVES:** 6
PREPARATION TIME: 15 minutes

If you wish *to double the batch, you have two options: bake and then freeze until ready for use, or freeze dough and thaw at room temperature for two to four hours and roll out as directed for a fresher product.*

> 2 cups whole wheat flour
> ³/₄ cup butter
> 1 teaspoon baking soda
> 1 teaspoon cream of tartar
> ¹/₃ cup frozen apple juice concentrate, thawed
> 1 egg
> 2 tablespoons hot water

◆ Preheat oven to 350°F. Place flour in large bowl. Cut in butter until it looks like little peas. Add baking soda, cream of tartar, apple juice concentrate, egg, and just enough water to make dough that can be rolled thin.

◆ Flour counter and roll out dough as thinly as possible. Cut into 4-inch squares with pizza wheel. Bake on baking sheet lined with parchment paper or foil in 350°F oven for 15 minutes, or until crackers start to brown at edges, watching carefully to remove end crackers as they brown if center ones are still soft.

◆ Pull parchment paper off baking sheet and let crackers cool completely. Store in air-tight container up to 2 weeks. Place sheet of paper towel in container to absorb any moisture that may make these crackers soft.

Chewy Biscotti

MAKES: 12   SERVES: 12
PREPARATION TIME: 20 minutes

You have a *choice here on whether to make these soft like a cake or crunchy like a cookie.*

1¼ cups dates, finely chopped
1 cup frozen apple juice concentrate, thawed
¼ cup canola oil
2 egg whites
1 teaspoon vanilla extract
1 cup whole wheat flour
½ cup wheat germ
1½ teaspoon baking powder
2 teaspoons ground cinnamon

◆ In saucepan, bring dates and apple juice concentrate to boil. Remove from heat and let cool for 10 minutes. Stir in oil and let cool to room temperature, at least 1 hour. (You can speed this up by placing in fridge.)

◆ Preheat oven to 350°F. In metal bowl, beat egg whites until slightly frothy; stir into date mixture. Stir in vanilla. In mixing bowl, combine flour, wheat germ, baking powder, and cinnamon; stir in date mixture just until combined.

◆ Rub loaf pan with butter; pour in batter. Bake in 350°F oven 45 to 50 minutes, until toothpick comes out clean. Let cool slightly before removing from pan to wire rack. Let cool completely; slice into twelve sticks.

◆ To make into more traditional biscotti, lay the slices on a greased baking sheet and bake in a preheated 325°F oven for 15 minutes until crisp.

TIP

AS A SPECIAL treat, dip the crispy biscotti in melted chocolate. Simply melt 4 ounces bittersweet chocolate in top of double boiler and stir in 2 tablespoons butter. Dip one end of the biscotti into the warm chocolate and then place on a baking sheet covered with foil. Allow to cool, and peel the cookies off the baking sheet. These are great for a holiday buffet or teacher's gift.

Banana Boats

Top these with *vanilla ice cream or lemon sorbet for special occasions.*

    4 bananas
    2 tablespoons carob or chocolate chips
    2 tablespoons miniature marshmallows

◆ Preheat oven or toaster oven to 450°F, or heat barbecue grill. Slit bananas lengthwise but not all the way through. Sprinkle carob chips and marshmallows evenly in each banana cavity. Wrap well in foil.

◆ Bake in 450°F oven or toaster oven, or place on barbecue grill for 15 to 20 minutes, until marshmallows and chips are melted.

Granola Bars

MAKES: 12 SERVES: 12
PREPARATION TIME: 20 minutes

These are a *great afterschool snack, filled with complex carbs and protein. The addition of raisins and/or chocolate chips makes an easier sell.*

    1 cup rolled oats
    1 cup slivered almonds
    2/3 cup packed brown sugar
    2/3 cup seedless raisins (optional)
    1/4 cup whole wheat flour
    1/4 cup chocolate chips (optional)
    1 tablespoon brewer's yeast
    2 teaspoons ground cinnamon
    1/2 teaspoon grated nutmeg
    1/2 cup butter

◆ Preheat oven to 375°F. In bowl, stir together rolled oats, almonds, brown sugar, raisins if desired, flour, chocolate chips if desired, brewer's yeast, cinnamon, and nutmeg. Melt butter in microwave oven for 30 to 45 seconds; stir into mixture.

◆ Firmly press mixture onto foil-lined baking sheet. (It will fill pan only halfway so scrunch up remaining foil to hold mixture in place.) Bake on top rack of 375°F oven for about 20 minutes, until browned and bubbling. Let cool for 2 to 4 minutes, or until sound of bubbling stops. Cut into squares or bars while still hot. Store in airtight container for up to 3 weeks.

Q-Bix

MAKES: 16 **SERVES:** 8
PREPARATION TIME: 15 minutes

This no-bake *snack does not travel well but is great for breakfast. A glass of milk and a couple Q-bix is all you need to send children off for the day with enough protein, dairy, and whole-grain carbs to last them until lunch.*

> ½ **cup almond butter**
> ⅓ **cup rolled oats**
> ¼ **cup dry milk powder**
> ¼ **cup shredded coconut**
> ¼ **cup wheat germ**
> ¼ **cup frozen apple juice concentrate, thawed**
> 2 **tablespoons seedless raisins (optional)**
> ½ **teaspoon ground cinnamon**
> ¼ **cup cocoa powder (optional)**

◆ In large bowl, thoroughly combine almond butter, rolled oats, milk powder, coconut, wheat germ, apple juice, raisins if desired, and cinnamon. Shape into sixteen 1-inch cubes. Measure cocoa powder into bowl and drop cubes in one at a time to coat.

◆ Place on baking sheet or baking pan and chill thoroughly before serving, at least 1 hour. Store in airtight container in refrigerator.

Sticky Rice Pudding

SERVES: 8
PREPARATION TIME: 10 minutes

This pudding calls *for short-grain brown rice, which can be found in the health food section at the grocery store, most health food stores, or Asian markets.*

¾ cup short-grain brown rice
1½ cups water
1 cup milk
½ cup golden raisins
½ cup liquid honey
1 tablespoon ground cinnamon

◆ In very large pot, mix rice with water; bring to boil. Reduce heat and simmer for 45 to 55 minutes, until rice is tender. Turn off heat. Add milk, raisins, honey, and cinnamon; let stand for 15 to 30 minutes to absorb milk. Serve warm with sprinkle of cinnamon. Store in fridge no longer than 48 hours

Vanilla Almond Shake

SERVES: 2
PREPARATION TIME: 3 minutes

*T*his **tasty shake** *is loaded with "good fats" and calories that will make up for any skipped meal.*

2 cups vanilla soy milk
½ cup silken tofu
¼ cup ice cubes
1 tablespoon almond butter
1 ripe banana
1 tablespoon ground flaxseed

◆ In blender, blend together soy milk, tofu, ice, almond butter, banana, and flaxseed for 3 to 5 minutes until smooth and thick like a milkshake.

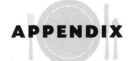

MAKE-AHEAD MIXES
AND SALAD DRESSINGS

We have come to rely on packaged mixes to make our weeknight suppers faster, but nothing could be simpler to prepare at home with healthier, fresher, less-expensive ingredients. Our homemade Cheese Coating is great to use for chicken fingers, or for baked vegetables or potatoes. Salad dressings, too, can be made better and less expensively at home. Here are some mix and dressing ideas that can be made ahead and stored in tightly lidded jars or zip-top bags in the fridge or cupboard. Kids love to mix these ingredients and my cooking class kids have invented variations that have surprised and delighted all of us.

Chile Spice

Use this mix by the teaspoonful to spice up any dish that is bland enough for the kids but needs a little zip for more grown-up tastebuds. It is great in tomato sauce or in our biscuit mix.

½ cup chile powder
¼ cup Mrs. Dash seasoning
8 teaspoons ground cumin
4 teaspoons dried oregano

4 teaspoons onion powder
2 teaspoons garlic powder
1 teaspoons cayenne pepper

◆ Mix together chile powder, Mrs. Dash, cumin, oregano, onion powder, garlic powder, and cayenne. Store in airtight container for up to 3 months.

Cheese Coating

U*se to coat chicken, zucchini cubes, or chopped sweet potatoes.*

4 cups dry whole wheat bread crumbs
1 cup dried parsley
¾ cup grated Parmesan cheese
½ cup olive oil

1 teaspoon garlic powder
1 teaspoon salt
1 teaspoon pepper

◆ Mix together bread crumbs, parsley, cheese, oil, garlic powder, salt, and pepper. Refrigerate in airtight container for up to 4 weeks or freeze up to 8 weeks. Coat chosen food in mixture; lay on baking sheet. Bake in preheated 400°F oven until cooked through. (Veggies need 10 to15 minutes; chicken may need 40.)

Whole Wheat Biscuit Mix

G*reat for last-minute biscuits to go with any meal!*

4 cups whole wheat flour
2 cups unbleached flour
1½ cups skim milk powder
1 cup granulated sugar

¾ cup wheat germ
½ cup plus 2 tablespoons baking powder
1 tablespoon salt
1½ cups butter

◆ In bowl, mix together whole wheat and unbleached flours, milk powder, sugar, wheat germ, baking powder, and salt; cut in butter. Store in fridge up to 3 weeks.
◆ Stir 2 cups of mix with 1 egg and mix in just enough water to make sticky dough. Drop by rounded spoonfuls onto baking sheet; bake for 10 to 25 minutes in preheated 375°F oven. Makes about 60 biscuits.

TIPS

ADD DIFFERENT LIQUIDS such as apple juice or buttermilk instead of water.

Stir in some Chile Spice and cornmeal to make cornmeal muffins.

Stir in extra milk and one egg and use as a pancake mix; be sure to thin it out considerably.

Add a handful of rolled oats and a mashed banana, and bake as muffins in muffin tins.

Sesame Topping

Use to add a crunchy twist to any meal. Sprinkle into a salad and use our Asian Dressing. Top any stir-fry to add some crunch and fiber. Sprinkle into soups instead of crackers. Serve as is for a great snack alternative to chips or popcorn.

2 cups rolled oats	1/3 cup sesame seeds
1/2 cup melted butter	1/4 cup garlic powder
1/3 cup shredded sharp Cheddar cheese	

◆ In bowl, combine oats, butter, cheese, sesame seeds, and garlic powder; spread on baking sheet. Bake in preheated 350°F oven for 15 minutes, or until lightly browned. Store in refrigerator up to 2 months.

Asian Dressing

1/2 cup canola oil	2 tablespoons lemon juice
2 tablespoons toasted sesame oil	2 tablespoons rice vinegar
1 tablespoon sesame seeds	1 teaspoon grated gingerroot

◆ In jar, shake together canola oil, sesame oil, sesame seeds, lemon juice, vinegar, ginger, and lemon rind. Refrigerate up to 1 month.

Italian Dressing

1 teaspoon lemon zest
½ cup extra-virgin olive oil
2 tablespoons balsamic vinegar
2 tablespoons red wine vinegar
1 tablespoon Dijon mustard
1 tablespoon light mayonnaise
1 teaspoon dried Italian herb seasoning (or any combination of basil, oregano, thyme leaves)
1 teaspoon garlic salt
Pepper to taste

◆ In jar, shake together lemon zest, oil, balsamic vinegar, red wine vinegar, mustard, mayonnaise, herb seasoning, garlic salt, and pepper. Refrigerate up to 1 month.

Mexican Dressing

This recipe is low in fat and is great as a dip for corn chips and for Mexican taco salad.

½ cup salsa
2 tablespoons red wine vinegar
2 tablespoons extra-virgin olive oil
1 tablespoon chopped fresh cilantro
1 teaspoon dried oregano
1 clove garlic, minced

◆ In jar, shake together salsa, vinegar, oil, cilantro, oregano, and garlic. Refrigerate up to 2 weeks.

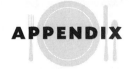

APPENDIX

QUICKIE MEALS
FROM WHAT YOU'VE GOT

Hᴇʀᴇ ᴀʀᴇ ꜱᴏᴍᴇ fast supper-savers and sides from your fridge, freezer, and pantry.

		PANTRY MEALS AND SIDES			
TO MAKE	USE	PLUS	IN A	FOR	TO SERVE WITH
Garlicky White Beans	1 (19-ounce) can white kidney beans, drained	1 tablespoon olive oil 1 clove garlic, minced 1/4 cup grated Parmesan cheese	skillet	4 min	barbecued chicken, beef, or pork
Taco Filling	1 (19-ounce) can refried beans	1/2 cup salsa	microwave oven (high)	3 min	salad and warmed taco shells
Lentil Soup	1 (19-ounce) can lentils, drained	1 (14-ounce) can chicken stock 1 cup frozen corn niblets	pot	5 min	bread and cheese
Chickpea Salad	1 (19-ounce) can chickpeas, drained	2 tablespoons olive oil 2 tablespoons lime juice 1 cup chopped fresh parsley leftover cooked rice	bowl	10 min	barbecued fish or chicken
Pad Thai	1 cup chopped peanuts	1/4 cup peanut sauce 1/4 cup light coconut milk 1/4 cup water 2 cups beansprouts	pot	5 min	4 cups cooked egg noodles

PANTRY SNACKS

TO MAKE	USE	PLUS	IN A	FOR	TO SERVE WITH
Mexican Tomato Soup	baked corn tortilla chips	1 (28-ounce) can pureed tomatoes 1 teaspoon garlic powder 1 teaspoon dried oregano 1/4 cup grated Parmesan cheese	pot	5 min	crackers and crudités
Brie Crackers	rye crackers	caramelized onions Brie cheese, sliced apple slices	broiler	3 min	cocktails
Cream Cheese Bites	rye crackers	cream cheese carrots, grated black olives	broiler	2 min	cocktails
Sweet Pecan Topping	2 cups chopped pecans	1/4 cup butter, melted 1/4 cup packed brown sugar	cookie sheet in 400°F oven	15 min	over mashed sweet potatoes or ice cream

PANTRY DESSERTS

TO MAKE	USE	PLUS	IN A	FOR
Fruit Cake	1 cup sliced almonds	1 package vanilla cake mix 1 cup raisins 1 cup applesauce 2 apples, sliced	cake pan	as directed
Cherry Trifle	1 (19-ounce) can cherry pie filling	1 (19-ounce) can vanilla pudding 3 cups cubed angel food cake	serving bowl	5 min
Pumpkin Pudding	1 (19-ounce) can pure pumpkin	2 eggs 1 cup packed brown sugar 1 cup evaporated milk	greased pie plate in in 425°F oven	1 hour

TO MAKE	USE	PLUS	IN A	FOR	TO SERVE WITH
Shrimp Sauté	4 cups frozen shrimp, thawed	1 tablespoon olive oil 2 cloves garlic, minced 2 cups frozen peas 1/4 cup dried parsley 1 cup chicken stock	skillet	10 min	salad and steamed rice
Seafood Marinara	2 cups frozen shrimp, thawed	1 (19-ounce) can tomato sauce 1/2 cup grated Parmesan cheese	skillet	8 min	linguine and salad
Curried Scallops	3 cups frozen scallops, thawed	1/4 cup butter 1 tablespoon curry powder 1 cup chopped frozen spinach	skillet	10 min	basmati rice
Spicy Puttanesca Sauce	1 cup extra-lean ground beef (thawed in microwave)	1 clove garlic, minced 1 (19-ounce can) spaghetti sauce 3 tablespoons anchovy paste 3 tablespoons capers 2 tablespoons olive tapenade 1 teaspoon hot pepper flakes	skillet	20 min	fusilli or spaghetti

FRIDGE MEALS AND SIDES

TO MAKE	USE	PLUS	IN A	FOR	TO SERVE WITH
Brunch Frittata	6 eggs	any leftover meat or cooked veggies	skillet in oven	20 min	bread and salad
Coleslaw	1 pound grated cabbage	¼ cup light mayonnaise 1 tablespoon sugar 2 tablespoons vinegar	bowl	2 min	barbecued anything
Stir-fried Cabbage	1 pound grated cabbage	1 tablespoon toasted sesame oil ¼ cup soy sauce 1 tablespoon grated gingerroot	skillet	5 min	burgers
Chicken Stir-fry	1 pound grated cabbage	3 boneless skinless chicken breasts, sliced 1 tablespoon toasted sesame oil ¼ cup soy sauce 1 tablespoon grated gingerroot	skillet	15 min	steamed rice

FRIDGE DESSERTS

TO MAKE	USE	PLUS	IN A	FOR
Warm Parfait	2 cups vanilla yogurt	3 cups frozen berries	microwave oven (high)	4 min
Fancy Parfait	3 cups suet-free mincemeat	8 vanilla wafers 3 cups frozen yogurt	freezer, layered into 4 martini glasses	1 to 8 hours

APPENDIX

NUTRITIONAL ANALYSES

THE ANALYSES LISTED here approximate and are per serving. Each recipe has been divided by the total number of servings, which includes both entrée and leftover portions, so to obtain the most accurate analysis be sure to divide each recipe as specified. Please note that analyses for Second Suppers and Grab & Go Lunches are not provided since they rely heavily on reserved amounts from previous recipes and each household will differ in how they choose to handle this.

I always prefer homemade or frozen stock that has a negligible nutrition profile and very low sodium count. In light of this, all recipes that call for stock have been analyzed using a one-to-one mixture of canned stock and water—the sodium levels in these analyses are very high. The idea was to provide a worst-case scenario in the salt counts; should you opt for canned stock, you will at least have a better picture of the nutrient value. Choosing homemade or frozen stock will result in a much lower sodium count than those given here.

Asian Sprout and Red Pepper Salad: Calories 80, Fat 7g, Carbohydrates 4g, Fiber 1g, Protein 2g, Sodium 33mg

Asparagus in Its Own Juices: Calories 77, Fat 6g, Carbohydrates 6g, Fiber 2g, Protein 2g, Sodium 270mg

Athenian Lamb and Lima Beans: Calories 329, Fat 10g, Carbohydrates 38g, Fiber 7g, Protein 26g, Sodium 760mg

Baked Mashed Potatoes and Potato Skins: Calories 233, Fat 8g, Carbohydrates 36g, Fiber 5g, Protein 6g, Sodium 202mg

Baked Pork Tenderloin with Spinach and Blue Cheese: Calories 344, Fat 14g, Carbohydrates 11g, Fiber 5g, Protein 43g, Sodium 595mg

Balsamic Barley Salad: Calories 256, Fat 7g, Carbohydrates 42g, Fiber 8g, Protein 10g, Sodium 405mg

Banana Boats: Calories 143, Fat 3g, Carbohydrates 32g, Fiber 3g, Protein 2g, Sodium 3mg

Beef Tenderloin Steaks with Peppercorn Rub: Calories 423, Fat 29g, Carbohydrates 15g, Fiber 3g, Protein 26g, Sodium 677mg

Better Spaghetti Sauce: Calories 279, Fat 13g, Carbohydrates 19g, Fiber 5g, Protein 14g, Sodium 605mg

Bistro Burgers: Calories 405, Fat 21g, Carbohydrates 17g, Fiber 4g, Protein 27g, Sodium 397mg

Black Bean Nachos: Calories 592, Fat 20g, Carbohydrates 78g, Fiber 18g, Protein 31g, Sodium 626mg

Boston Baked Beans: Calories 282, Fat 3g, Carbohydrates 52g, Fiber 15g, Protein 14g, Sodium 125mg

Celery Peanut Butter Logs: Calories 190, Fat 16g, Carbohydrates 7g, Fiber 2g, Protein 8g, Sodium 159mg

Chewy Biscotti: Calories 186, Fat 5g, Carbohydrates 34g, Fiber 4g, Protein 4g, Sodium 55mg

Chicken Breasts with Spicy Rub: Calories 424, Fat 24g, Carbohydrates 13g, Fiber 1g, Protein 39g, Sodium 705mg

Chicken Cacciatore: Calories 358, Fat 12g, Carbohydrates 27g, Fiber 5g, Protein 36g, Sodium 1,368 mg

Chicken Soup (using canned stock and water): Calories 136, Fat 1g, Carbohydrates 15g, Fiber 3g, Protein 14g, Sodium 2,223 mg

Chicken Stuffed with Sun-Dried Tomatoes and Chèvre: Calories 372, Fat 11g, Carbohydrates 39g, Fiber 8g, Protein 37g, Sodium 1,548mg

Creamy Baked Salmon: Calories 177, Fat 4g, Carbohydrates 7g, Fiber 0g, Protein 27g, Sodium 275mg

Crisp Topping: Calories 227, Fat 13g, Carbohydrates 26g, Fiber 2g, Protein 4g, Sodium 86mg

Crustless Broccoli and Cheese Quiches: Calories 390, Fat 29g, Carbohydrates 14g, Fiber 1g, Protein 19g, Sodium 438mg

Cucumber Faces: Calories 60, Fat 3g, Carbohydrates 7g, Fiber 2g, Protein 3g, Sodium 89 mg

Easy Minestrone: Calories 271, Fat 8g, Carbohydrates 41g, Fiber 10g, Protein 12g, Sodium 918mg

Five-Spice Chicken with Hot Slaw: Calories 379, Fat 10g, Carbohydrates 23g, Fiber 3g, Protein 50g, Sodium 1,427mg

Granola Bars: Calories 254, Fat 15g, Carbohydrates 30g, Fiber 3g, Protein 4g, Sodium 86mg

Grilled Vegetable Soup (using canned stock and water): Calories 383, Fat 23g, Carbohydrates 23g, Fiber 4g, Protein 21g, Sodium 3,179mg

Guacamole: Calories 177, Fat 16g, Carbohydrates 11g, Fiber 4g, Protein 3g, Sodium 26mg

Homemade Chicken Fingers: Calories 233, Fat 6g, Carbohydrates 14g, Fiber 1g, Protein 28g, Sodium 393mg

Jamaican-ish Pork: Calories 183, Fat 6g, Carbohydrates 2g, Fiber 1g, Protein 29g, Sodium 240mg

Lasagne Roll-Ups: Calories 645, Fat 13g, Carbohydrates 98g, Fiber 7g, Protein 34g, Sodium 978mg

Lemony Baked Shrimp: Calories 372, Fat 10g, Carbohydrates 20g, Fiber 1g, Protein 49g, Sodium 779mg

Lemony Steamed Broccoli: Calories 9, Fat 0g, Carbohydrates 1g, Fiber 1g, Protein 1g, Sodium 51mg

Lower-Fat Chili con Carne: Calories 423, Fat 13g, Carbohydrates 55g, Fiber 21g, Protein 26g, Sodium 381mg

Meat Loaf Florentine with Salsa: Calories 391, Fat 24g, Carbohydrates 18g, Fiber 3g, Protein 26g, Sodium 811mg

Molasses Lentil Soup (using canned stock and water): Calories 359, Fat 5g, Carbohydrates 52g, Fiber 18g, Protein 27g, Sodium 2,203mg

Oatmeal Cookies: Calories 181, Fat 7g, Carbohydrates 28g, Fiber 1g, Protein 3g, Sodium 128mg

Oh Mega Crackers: Calories 48, Fat 2g, Carbohydrates 6g, Fiber 1g, Protein 2g, Sodium 190mg

Parmesan Barley Risotto (using canned stock and water): Calories 208, Fat 3g, Carbohydrates 35g, Fiber 7g, Protein 9g, Sodium 1,733mg

Parsnip Puree Chicken Stew (using canned stock and water): Calories 360, Fat 11g, Carbohydrates 42g, Fiber 9g, Protein 24g, Sodium 973mg

Poppy Seed Noodles: Calories 118, Fat 5g, Carbohydrates 15g, Fiber 1g, Protein 3g, Sodium 5mg

Pork Roast Dijon: Calories 599, Fat 29g, Carbohydrates 36g, Fiber 5g, Protein 40g, Sodium 263mg

Pumpkin Pie: Calories 128, Fat 2g, Carbohydrates 25g, Fiber 3g, Protein 5g, Sodium 54mg

Q-Bix: Calories 181, Fat 12g, Carbohydrates 16g, Fiber 3g, Protein 6g, Sodium 21mg

Quick and Delicious Peanut Butter Cookies: Calories 177, Fat 11g, Carbohydrates 16g, Fiber 1g, Protein 6g, Sodium 108mg

Quick Italian Sausage and Kidney Bean Soup (using canned stock and water): Calories 271, Fat 6g,

Carbohydrates 41g, Fiber 13g, Protein 13g, Sodium 2,215mg

Quinoa and Carrots (made with water): Calories 209, Fat 5g, Carbohydrates 35g, Fiber 5g, Protein 6g, Sodium 79mg

Red Pepper Rice: Calories 181, Fat 2g, Carbohydrates 37g, Fiber 1g, Protein 4g, Sodium 367mg

Rice with Grated Carrots (using canned stock and water): Calories 197, Fat 2g, Carbohydrates 39g, Fiber 2g, Protein 4g, Sodium 1,087mg

Roast Beef with Rosemary and Garlic Veggies: Calories 220, Fat 9g, Carbohydrates 6g, Fiber 1g, Protein 26g, Sodium 333mg

Roasted Chicken to Please Everybody (with skin): Calories 560, Fat 31g, Carbohydrates 30g, Fiber 4g, Protein 36g, Sodium 386mg

Roasted Vegetables with Garlic Oil: Calories 131, Fat 5g, Carbohydrates 20g, Fiber 5g, Protein 4g, Sodium 150mg

Salmon Cakes with Caper Mayo: Calories 365, Fat 15g, Carbohydrates 29g, Fiber 2g, Protein 28g, Sodium 837mg

Salmon with Spinach and Feta in Parchment: Calories 325, Fat 17g, Carbohydrates 12g, Fiber 5g, Protein 36g, Sodium 815mg

Scallops and Soybeans in Sake Stock (using canned stock and water): Calories 372, Fat 13g, Carbohydrates 10g, Fiber 6g, Protein 32g, Sodium 980mg

Sesame Broccoli Salad: Calories 68, Fat 6g, Carbohydrates 3g, Fiber 1g, Protein 2g, Sodium 307mg

Sesame Fish Cakes with Baby Bok Choy: Calories 400, Fat 3g, Carbohydrates 56g, Fiber 6g, Protein 39g, Sodium 2,542 mg

Slow-Cooked Beer-Braised Beef: Calories 541, Fat 36g, Carbohydrates 9g, Fiber 1g, Protein 37g, Sodium 207mg

Southwestern Fish Sticks: Calories 253, Fat 4g, Carbohydrates 27g, Fiber 2g, Protein 27g, Sodium 502mg

Souvlaki Pork with Tossed Greek Salad: Calories 275, Fat 15g, Carbohydrates 8g, Fiber 1g, Protein 28g, Sodium 234mg

Spicy Asian Salad: Calories 107, Fat 6g, Carbohydrates 14g, Fiber 2g, Protein 3g, Sodium 16mg

Steamed Dilly Carrots: Calories 52, Fat 1g,

Carbohydrates 12g, Fiber 3g, Protein 1g, Sodium 573mg

Steamed Snow Peas: Calories 27, Fat 0g, Carbohydrates 5g, Fiber 1g, Protein 1g, Sodium 2mg

Sticky Rice Pudding: Calories 181, Fat 2g, Carbohydrates 41g, Fiber 1g, Protein 3g, Sodium 19mg

Sunday Ham with Potatoes: Calories 520, Fat 31g, Carbohydrates 23g, Fiber 2g, Protein 38g, Sodium 231mg

Sunday Ham Soup with Romano Beans and Kale: Calories 155, Fat 5g, Carbohydrates 18g, Fiber 3g, Protein 10g, Sodium 532mg

Sweet Potato Muffins: Calories 219, Fat 9g, Carbohydrates 34g, Fiber 2g, Protein 3g, Sodium 201mg

Thai Stuffed Pork with Mashed Apples and Squash: Calories 427, Fat 14g, Carbohydrates 30g, Fiber 3g, Protein 43g, Sodium 170mg

Tofu Caesar Salad: Calories 39, Fat 3g, Carbohydrates 2g, Fiber 1g, Protein 3g, Sodium 30mg

Tuna Sailboats: Calories 282, Fat 12g, Carbohydrates 31g, Fiber 5g, Protein 16g, Sodium 503mg

Vanilla Almond Shake: Calories 302, Fat 18g, Carbohydrates 26g, Fiber 8g, Protein 16g, Sodium 45mg

Veggies, Week 2: Calories 58, Fat 0g, Carbohydrates 12g, Fiber 4g, Protein 3g, Sodium 19mg

Veggies, Week 4: Calories 124, Fat 1g, Carbohydrates 29g, Fiber 9g, Protein 4g, Sodium 88mg

Whole Wheat Graham Crackers: Calories 309, Fat 17g, Carbohydrates 36g, Fiber 5g, Protein 7g, Sodium 381mg

Zucchini Muffins: Calories 221, Fat 9g, Carbohydrates 32g, Fiber 2g, Protein 4g, Sodium 192mg

As analyzed with Sierra MasterCook program and rounded to the nearest whole number.

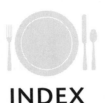

INDEX